Clinical Thermology

Subseries Thermotherapy

M. Gautherie (Ed.)

Whole Body Hyperthermia: Biological and Clinical Aspects

With Contributions by
H. I. Robins · J. D. Cohen · A. J. Neville

With 43 Figures and 9 Tables

Springer-Verlag
Berlin Heidelberg New York
London Paris Tokyo
Hong Kong Barcelona
Budapest

Dr. Michel Gautherie
Laboratoire de Thermologie Biomédicale
Université Louis Pasteur
Institut National de la Santé
et de la Recherche Médicale
11, rue Humann
67085 Strasbourg Cedex, France

Justin D. Cohen, M.D.
Division of Hematology
and Oncology
University of Colorado
Health Sciences Center
4200 East 9th Avenue
Denver, Colorado 80262
USA

H. Ian Robins, M.D., Ph. D.
University of Wisconsin
Clinical Cancer Center
Department of Human Oncology
600 Highland Avenue
Madison, WI 53792, USA

Alan J. Neville, M.D.
The Ontario Cancer Foundation
11 Concession Street
Hamilton, Ontario L8V 1C3
Canada

ISBN 3-540-54560-3 Springer-Verlag Berlin Heidelberg NewYork
ISBN 0-387-54560-3 Springer-Verlag NewYork Berlin Heidelberg

Library of Congress Cataloging-in-Publication Data
Whole body hyperthermia: biological and clinical aspects / M. Gautherie (ed.); with contributions by H.I. Robins, J.D. Cohen, A.J. Neville. p. cm. – (Clinical thermology. Subseries thermotherapy) Includes bibliographical references and index.
ISBN 3-540-54560-3 (alk. paper). – ISBN 0-387-54560-3 (alk. paper)
1. Thermotherapy. I. Gautherie, Michel. II. Robins, H.I. (H. Ian) III. Cohen, J.D. (Justin D.) IV. Neville, A.J. (Alan J.) [DNLM: 1. Hyperthermia, Induced. WB 469 W628] RM865.W46 1992 615.8'32 – dc20 DNLM/DLC
91-5219

Printed in Germany

Typesetting: K+V Fotosatz GmbH, Beerfelden
Printing and binding: K. Triltsch, Graphischer Betrieb, Würzburg
27/3145-5 4 3 2 1 0 – Printed on acid-free paper

Albert Szent-Gyorgyi described discovery as seeing what everyone else has seen and thinking what nobody else has thought. In this sense Dr. Thomas E. Davis is a true discoverer. His excellence as a teacher, clinician and cancer researcher has served as an inspiration to the authors with regard to the practice of clinical oncology and the pursuit of many of the investigations described in this text.

Contents

Acknowledgement

The authors gratefully acknowledge the editorial and technical support of Cindy Schmitt, Bonnie Rayho, and Kathy Edge.

1 Introduction

1.1 Background

Anticancer effects of elevated (noncauterizing) temperature were first observed in ancient Egyptian times (Oleson and Dewhirst 1983). Hippocrates (460 – 377 B.C.) later incorporated fever therapy into a homeopathic approach to disease (i.e., treating a disease with a symptom of that disease). In the fourth century, Refus of Ephesus advocated the use of fever induction to treat malignant diseases (Kluger 1980). In the nineteenth century tumor regressions accompanying high fevers were reported both by Busch and Bruns (Busch 1866; Bruns 1888). At the end of the nineteenth century, Coley reported an anecdotal series of cancer patients who responded to fevers induced by erysipelas and bacterial endotoxins (Coley 1893; Nauts et al. 1953). In 1935, Warren induced "artificial fevers" using diathermy in conjunction with incandescent light bulbs and also described antineoplastic activity (Warren 1935).

The hypothetical basis for using hyperthermia as cancer therapy by these early clinical workers can, at best, be described as intuitive. A more comprehensive review of the early history of hyperthermia can be found elsewhere (Meyer 1984b). During the past two decades, however, a formidable accumulation of laboratory data has provided a sound rationale for incorporating hyperthermia into modern cancer therapy. The potential therapeutic impact of hyperthermia has not yet been clearly defined.

Neoplastic disease processes are now recognized as being heterogenous with various cell subpopulations having different sensitivities to any given therapy. Thus, both clinical and preclinical investigators are currently pursuing treatment strategies which incorporate a multimodality approach to maximize the chances of killing all tumor cell subpopulations (Robins 1984). In this regard, it is the central theme of this text to show that whole body hyperthermia (WBH) may serve as a useful adjunct to radiation and/or drugs in the development of curative therapies for neoplastic diseases which are currently refractory to conventional therapy. All aspects of both preclinical and clinical WBH, ranging from molecular biology and physiology to WBH methodologies and clinical trials, will be comprehensively reviewed. It is our intention to provide the reader with a definitive resource to evaluate the current status and future potential of WBH. In so doing, we will attempt to present the various perspectives and insights derived from the efforts of investigators throughout the world. We hope this will encourage an expanded investigative commitment to this exciting and innovative approach to cancer therapy.

The first scientific rationale for the potential of hyperthermia as a cancer treatment modality was derived from the observations that some classes of cancer cells were sensitive to temperatures in excess of 41 °C. Although certain examples of neoplastic cells are more sensitive to heat than are their normal cell counterparts, the literature in this regard is limited (Chen and Heidelberger 1969; Giovanella et al. 1973; Karnovsky 1967; Kase and Hahn 1976; Robins et al. 1983d, 1988c; Schrek 1966). Thus, the generalization that neoplastic cells are uniquely thermal sensitive is not clearly valid. In selected settings, however, a case has been made for exploiting the thermal sensitivities of leukemias and lymphomas (Robins et al. 1984b), as well as some solid tumors such as primary brain tumors (Ibuchi et al. 1988).

Hyperthermia in general, and WBH in particular, should be used as adjuncts to other forms of cancer therapy. We have long been skeptical about the clinical utility of WBH as a single modality. WBH alone yields low response rates, as well as short response durations in the treatment of spontaneous neoplasms (Bull et al. 1979a; Dewhirst et al. 1982; Manning et al. 1982; Marmor et al. 1979b; Oleson and Dewhirst 1983; Robins 1984; Robins and Neville 1986; Robins et al. 1985b). The potential biological basis for these observations is discussed in an insightful review by Oleson and Dewhirst (Dewhirst et al. 1982).

1.2 Systemic Versus Local and Regional Hyperthermia

The medical systems developed for clinical hyperthermia fall into three major categories: (1) local, (2) regional, and (3) systemic, or whole body.

Local hyperthermia can be accomplished with several different technologies (e.g., capacitive and inductive, radio frequency, ultrasound and microwave (Oleson and Dewhirst 1983; Oleson et al. 1984a; Streffer 1978; Nussbaum 1982; Hornback 1984; Stewart and Gibbs 1984; Hill 1982; Kim and Hahn 1979; LeVeen et al. 1976). Early clinical reports regarding the efficacy of local hyperthermia were anecdotal in nature. There were problems relating to thermometry and the use of study populations, which included patients with solitary lesions. Thus, data was lacking on response rates in matched tumors. However, controlled studies have recently been conducted which support the use of local hyperthermia in conjunction with radiotherapy (Arcangeli et al. 1983; Corry et al. 1982; Dewhirst et al. 1984; Kim et al. 1982; Marmor and Hahn 1980; Overgaard 1981a; Steeves et al. 1986).

Other problems with local hyperthermia have not been solved to date, including uneven tumor heating and the use of invasive thermometry. The uneven heating produced by current local hyperthermia technologies is a significant concern. The work of Oleson and Dewhirst supports the conclusion that (in patient groups treated with the specific equipment), it is the lowest temperature achieved in a tumor mass which is the best predictor of response (Dewhirst et al. 1984; Oleson et al. 1983; Oleson and Dewhirst 1983). In addition to such technical difficulties, there may be a conceptual problem relating to local hyperthermia: most cancers which are refractory to standard therapy are systemic diseases. Thus, local hyperthermia is usually limited to a palliative role. However, local hyperthermia may contribute to achieving cure in the treatment of some primary cancers (e.g., primary head and neck, cervical, and CNS cancers) which have limited potential to metastasize.

Deep regional hyperthermia has been hampered by the same technological limitations described for local hyperthermia; invasive thermometry and temperature homogeneity are more problematic. Existing technologies developed include electromagnetic induction heating by circumferential coil, microwave, and ultrasound (Baker et al. 1982; Lele and Parker 1982; Marmor 1983; Oleson 1982; Oleson and Dewhirst 1983; Oleson et al. 1983; Sapozink et al. 1984; Stewart et al. 1984; Storm et al. 1979a, b, 1981). Heating sessions (i.e., time-temperature profiles) accomplished with these regional systems are not reproducible for a given patient, let alone between patients, so that controlled randomized trials with regional hyperthermia are extremely difficult. Establishment of a specific anatomical site, e.g., the pelvis, in which there is more assured delivery of a given thermal dose may be the next challenge for workers in this area. In spite of the difficulties described for local and regional hyperthermia, their proponents point out that there is the potential for exceeding the temperature maximum of WBH (i.e., ~42 °C) in specific tissues.

It is relevant to this discussion to highlight the point that limb perfusion hyperthermia is performed with the same temperature limitations as WBH (Cavaliere et al. 1967; Janoff et al. 1982; Rege et al. 1983; Stehlin et al. 1975). Limb perfusion hyperthermia for the treatment of sarcomas and melanomas was first reported in 1967 by Cavaliere et al. and later by Stehlin et al. 1975. Impressive response rates were obtained when hyperthermia was combined with chemotherapy. These small studies were retrospective and relied on historal controls, so that they must be interpreted with caution. Nevertheless, some observers consider that these nonrandomized studies represent the most impressive historical argument for clinical hyperthermia (Oleson and Dewhirst 1983). A published prospective randomized trial done by Ghussen et al. (1984) in Germany demonstrates the efficacy of perfusional hyperthermia. Additional controlled multiinstitutional clinical trials of regional hyperthermia are currently in progress in Italy and Sweden.

For the purpose of this discussion, the reader should be cautioned that, at a minimum, anatomical considerations (in part relating to depth of heating) should dominate the decision making regarding local versus WBH. However, in contrasting the relative therapeutic merits of regional versus WBH, physiological considerations become dominant. By way of example, the use of regional hyperthermia to the area of the thorax to treat a lung cancer is not presently feasible (Robins et al. 1986a). Thus, WBH is most appropriate for this task. It should be further noted that the application of regional hyperthermia can result in systemic heating (Pilepich et al. 1987). In considering the relative merits of regional versus systemic hyperthermia, many have speculated on the potential for doing WBH with a regional boost (Atkinson 1979). For specific physiological considerations this is not readily feasible (Robins et al. 1983b), although the combination of WBH and local hyperthermia may be practical, as will be discussed later in Chap. 5.

In contrast to local and regional hyperthermia, WBH addresses the issue of distant metastases and, therefore, has potential as an adjunct to other therapies, directed at the cure of systemic malignancies. The variety of methodologies currently available for WBH (to be reviewed in detail in text to follow) reflects a lack of consensus on the part of clinicians as to the best application of physiological and physical principles for systemic hyperthermia. Controversies in the field of WBH include concerns relating to toxicity, the need for mechanical ventilation, labor intensive aspects, and the adequacy of the temperature reached. Details relating to these issues will be adequately reviewed so the reader can weigh their significance, and perhaps contrast them to the relative limitation now inherent in local and regional hyperthermia.

1.3 Conceptual Approaches to the Therapeutic Use of WBH

1.3.1 Drugs

Preclinical and clinical data have demonstrated that hyperthermia can potentiate the tumoricidal effects of chemotherapeutic agents (see Chap. 4). Thermal enhancement of drug cytotoxicity may have its greatest potential for therapeutic impact in the setting of WBH. Strategies for such combined modality therapy must address factors affecting therapeutic index, i.e., the relative toxicity of a therapy for neoplastic versus normal tissues. Outlined below are concepts which may prove relevant to WBH-chemotherapy clinical trials.

Most malignancies which require chemotherapy are systemic diseases. Combining therapy with systemic heating, i.e., WBH, is therefore a logical step in developing innovative and hopefully curative cancer therapies.

Conceptual approaches to the problem of bone marrow toxicity during WBH can take several forms. It has been shown that during the plateau phase of radiant heat WBH, marrow temperature is as much as 1 °C lower than core temperature (Hugander et al. 1987). Thus, for drugs with primarily myelosuppressive toxicity, such as carboplatin, therapeutic index may be increased by administering carboplatin specifically during the plateau phase of WBH. Such an approach is reasonable, particularly for patients free of marrow involvement.

Alternatively, one can utilize drugs whose major toxicity is myelosuppression, e.g., melphalan, carboplatin, or nitrosourea, with relative impunity in the setting of bone marrow transplantation (BMT) (Robins et al. 1984b, 1986b), as patients will be rescued from their toxicity by virtue of bone marrow transplant.

Although the use of WBH and chemotherapy in a metastatic setting may prove therapeutic, this combination may play a more significant role in an adjuvant setting. Here the term "adjuvant" refers to therapy directed at sterilizing micrometastases in patients who have been rendered free of all gross and detectable disease by surgery, but are at high risk for disease recurrence. (To avoid confusion, it is proposed that the term "adjunctive" be applied to situations in which hyperthermia is used to potentiate other forms of therapy). By way of example, adjuvant chemotherapy has both delayed disease recurrence, and increased survival of patients with stage II breast cancer, i.e. with axillary node involvement (Bonadonna and Valagussa 1981; Rossi et al. 1980). However, at least 33% of treated patients will relapse in 5 years with systemic disease (Bonadonna and Valagussa 1981; Rossi et al. 1980). Although relapse after adjuvant chemotherapy suggests drug resistance, interestingly, patients who have received adjuvant chemotherapy (and who subsequently developed metastatic disease) will respond to the same drugs that have been given in the adjuvant setting (Bitran et al. 1983; Rossi et al. 1980).

One explanation for these results, i.e., kinetic resistance, involves an inadequate microvasculature for drug delivery. Ironically, this comes at a time when the patients' tumor burdens are minimal and multidrug therapy should have its major impact. It is argued that WBH might help to overcome kinetic resistance (as opposed to biochemical resistance) by increasing membrane drug permeability, or by altering cellular metabolism and DNA repair capacity such that residual tumor cells become more sensitive to lower drug concentration. These theoretical proposals are testable in both transplantable and spontaneous animal models.

When one proposes adding WBH to adjuvant chemotherapy, the clinical feasibility of WBH becomes an important issue. In Chap. 5, methodologies appropriate to this task will be described.

Another novel approach is to use nonmyelosuppressive chemotherapeutic agents in combination with WBH, e.g., lonidamine (Silvestrini et al. 1983; Robins et al. 1988a). In a similar context, a group of drugs which for the sake of discussion will be termed "labilizers", are worthy of consideration. Labilizers are drugs that have no activity against neoplastic cells at normothermic temperatures but promote antineoplastic activity in the setting of hyperthermia. Anesthetic agents represent one class of drugs in this grouping (Clark et al. 1983; Robins et al. 1982; Robins et al. 1984a; Yatvin 1977; Yatvin et al. 1979, 1980; Yau 1979). It is significant that in animal models and in man such drugs can be administered safely (in doses which demonstrate antineoplastic activity in laboratory studies) in a temperature range consistent with WBH. To illustrate, the normal tissue toxicities of lidocaine and thiopental have been evaluated in both murine and porcine systems using the WBH temperature range of 41 °–42 °C (Robins 1984; Robins et al. 1991 a, b). These same drugs can potentially provide antineoplastic cell activity (Robins et al. 1984 a). At the Wisconsin Clinical Cancer Center, these drugs are given to patients in combination during WBH to provide sedation (Sorrell 1980) and for seizure and arrhythmia prophylaxis (Robins et al. 1985 b), as well as for their potential antineoplastic activity (Robins et al. 1984 a). We argue that such screening of drugs preclinically may lead to increased clinical efficacy as well as diminished toxicity. As suggested by others, research in the area of hyperthermia pharmacology is the key to optimizing WBH as a treatment modality (Kapp 1982).

To further optimize the design of clinical trials, both temperature and heat-drug sequencing should be studied preclinically in terms of both net cell kill and therapeutic index. Specifically, it should not be assumed that simultaneous drug-WBH administration or using the "highest" temperature will be optimal. By way of example: (a) Mini et al. (1986) have demonstrated that synergism between 5-fluorouracil (5-FU) and hyperthermia only occurs when 5-FU follows heat; (b) early results in a temperature range, i.e., ~40.5 °C, favor the drug-WBH arm reported by Englehardt in 1987; and (c) the optimal temperature for interferon and WBH is 40.5 °C (Robins 1984; Robins et al. 1989 b). Further, there may be scenarios in which simultaneous drug-WBH administration produces maximum neoplastic cell killing, but other sequences may produce an optimal ratio of neoplastic to normal cell kill.

1.3.2 Immunotherapy

As will be discussed in Chap. 2, the combination of WBH and various forms of immunotherapy, e.g., interferon, are actively undergoing preclinical (Groveman et al. 1984) and clinical investigation (Robins et al. 1989 b). Other research in this area is perhaps of a more speculative nature. For example, WBH may selectively enhance the immunogenicity of transformed cells in preclinical experimental systems (Hank et al. 1983). Thus, WBH might promote persistent antigenicity of residual leukemic cells in patients treated with allogenic BMT (Robins 1984; Robins et al. 1984 b). In such a case, WBH might enhance a graft versus leukemia reaction and decrease the chances of leukemic relapse. In addition, WBH may have a direct effect on the native immune system of a bone marrow transplant patient (i.e., immunosuppression) and thereby WBH may decrease host versus graft reactions (rejection) (Robins 1984; Robins et al. 1984 b). Early clinical data consistent with these postulates have been published (Robins et al. 1986 b).

1.3.3 Radiotherapy

The well-known cytoreductive advantages regarding the combination of hyperthermia and ionizing irradiation (Dewey et al. 1980) is fully discussed in Chap. 3. Less well recognized is the potential for WBH to attenuate the traditional toxicities of radiation to normal tissues. Figure 1 demonstrates the relationship of the effects of radiation on normal and neoplastic tissue. We believe there may be the potential to separate these curves. By way of example, in preliminary murine and human studies, Robins et al. (1990 b) have demonstrated the ability of WBH to attenuate the effects of radiation-induced thrombocytopenia associated with therapeutic total body irradiation (TBI). Similarly, preclinical studies consistent with this notion have been reported (Robins 1984; Steeves et al. 1987). These investigators have speculated that the enhancement of therapeutic index in these studies may relate to WBH-induced humoral factors resulting in the stimulation of hematopoietic cells production. (Thus, WBH may have potential to act as an exogenous inducer of hematopoietic stimulating factors.)

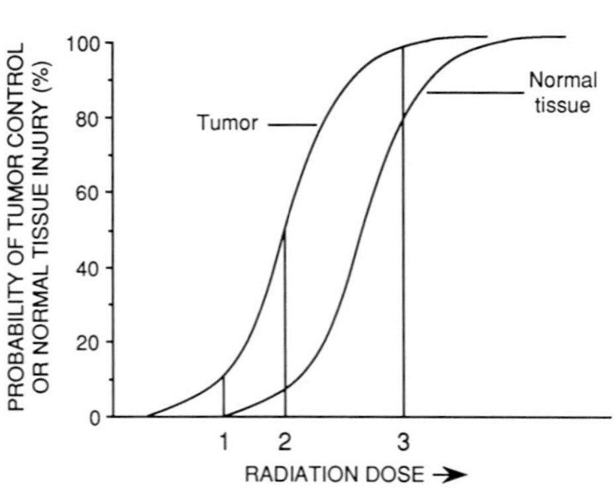

Fig. 1. Hypothetical relationships between three radiation doses and their relative effects on normal and neoplastic tissues. A theoretical effect of hyperthermia may relate to increasing the separation between these two curves, thereby permitting a greater tumor response rate for a given level of normal tissue injury

1.4 Summary

There is a preclinical rationale for WBH which is scientifically sound. Realizing the potential of WBH to be a useful form of cancer therapy requires further basic research and controlled clinical trials. It is in part the focus of this text to provide a foundation of knowledge to evaluate and initiate future studies. It is anticipated that a definitive evaluation of the efficacy of systemic hyperthermia as an adjunct to cancer treatment should occur during the next decade.

2 Hyperthermia and the Immune System

2.1 Introduction

Historically, immune and inflammatory responses associated with pyrexia have been implicated in host defenses against infection and neoplasia (Pettigrew and Ludgate 1977; Robins and Neville 1986). Early clinical studies by W.C. Coley, in the 1890s showed that significant tumor responses could be achieved by injecting bacterial filtrates into patients with advanced malignancy. Moreover, since some patients appeared to develop a tachyphylaxis to the pyrexia induced by the injected "toxins," the hypothesis arose that tumor destruction was not solely the result of the hyperthermic temperature achieved, but that the immune system of the patient was also involved (Nauts et al. 1953). The results of several animal studies performed in the first half of this century lent credence to this hypothesis and expanded it to suggest that hyperthermia-induced tumor cell damage stimulated the immune system to kill the remainder of the cancer (Westermark 1927; Johnson 1940).

What these studies failed to address, and what most subsequent in vivo and clinical hyperthermia studies have yet to answer, is the biological relevance of the immune system in the response of tumors to hyperthermia applied locally or systemically. Much of the research describing the immunobiology of hyperthermia has focused on the effects of elevated temperature in vitro, or in vivo, on isolated components of the immune system, either cellular or soluble mediators, or both. The wide diversity of animal tumor models employed (many using immunogenic transplantable tumors), as well as diverse heating modalities, temperatures, and heating times have produced a confusing amalgam of conflicting data. This presents the clinician interested in WBH with no firm guidelines as to how relevant the observed changes in the various immune parameters during hyperthermia may become for an individual patient undergoing WBH.

This chapter will describe the effects of elevated temperature on the multiple components of the immune system – including a summary of the literature describing the effects of clinical WBH on the immune system. Much of the data describing the immunological effects of hyperthermia derive from in vitro studies; while these data will be reviewed briefly, no attempt will be made to discuss, in detail, the in vitro methodology of these immunological assays or to re-

Table 1. Problematic issues surrounding hyperthermia immunobiology

General
In vitro vs in vivo studies
Effects on an immune pathway vs isolated components
Hyperthermia temperature employed; duration of heating; thermal dose
Variation in heating methodology; direct thermal effects vs nonthermal physical effects of the methodology employed
Relevance of immediate vs delayed and transient prolonged changes in immune function
Direct effect of heat on immune cells vs indirect effect via release of soluble mediators from other immune cells or from tumor cells
Species differences in immune system e.g., rat vs mouse vs hamster
Ability to discriminate between direct hyperthermia-induced tumor regression vs participation of the immune system
Hyperthermic induction of immune cells or soluble mediators vs facilitation of activity of pretreatment levels of such cells or mediators
Immunogenicity of the majority of transplantable animal tumors
Clinical WBH
Immune status of normal subjects vs cancer patients
In vitro assays performed at 37 °C on blood from patients during or after WBH vs in vitro assays performed at elevated temperatures
Effect of anesthesia on immune system of patients undergoing WBH
Possible significance of concurrent administration of antineoplastic drugs or biological response modifiers, e.g., interferons
Questionable therapeutic relevance of the manipulation of the immune system against most human cancers
End point analysis – difficulty in separating direct antitumor effects of hyperthermia from indirect effects via the immune system
Promotion or inhibition of tumor spread by WBH; the controversy surrounding WBH and metastasis

view exhaustively the basic concepts of tumor immunology save to mention, where appropriate, the difficulties in extrapolating to the clinical situation. Table 1 outlines a series of problems inherent in the interpretation of studies of the effects of hyperthermia on the immune system and several of these will be expanded on below.

2.2 In Vitro Studies of Hyperthermia and Immune Effector Cells

The potential clinical relevance of studying in vitro responses of individual immunological effector cells to elevated temperature remains uncertain. Historically, many different incubation temperatures and incubation times have been employed. The immunological parameters studied and the assays for testing them have often not been shown to be useful in assessing human antitumor immunity and it is therefore not clear whether increased activity during hyperthermia (or vice versa) would impact on response rates to clinical hyperthermia treatment. The discussion that follows focuses firstly on the direct effects of hyperthermia in vitro on B and T lymphocyte, monocyte-macrophage, and natural killer (NK) cell activity, and subsequently on the effects of a variety of biological response modifiers in combination with immunological effector cells during incubation at hyperthermic temperatures.

While reports of the effect of elevated temperature on lymphocyte subgroups are often contradictory, there seems to be some agreement that B cell number and function are either reduced or little affected by exposure for about 1 – 3 h in vitro to temperatures in the 37 °– 42 °C range (Onsrud 1983; Jampel et al. 1983). Onsrud showed, for example, that along with marginal effects on lymphocyte viability in cell populations from healthy human donors, there was nevertheless a significant reduction in the number of cells bearing Fc receptors for IgG. In contrast, there was only a slight reduction in sheep red cell rosetting (a T cell function) and this was restored to normal following incubation overnight at 37 °C.

Izumi et al. (1983) studied the in vivo effects of elevated temperatures on both human and murine lymphocytes. These investigators were investigating the clinical use of WBH in cancer patients (see Koga et al. 1983) and were concerned about a possible deleterious effect of WBH on the immune system. They noted little loss of lymphocyte viability at 39 °C (1 – 5 h water bath exposure-trypan blue dye exclusion test) but observed a time-dependent significant loss of viability at 42 °C. In both human and murine lymphocyte populations, 42 °C incubation inhibited phytohemagglutinin (PHA)-induced lymphocyte blastogenesis. Rosette formation was likewise reduced at 42 °C. Kalland and Dahlquist (1983) using normal human volunteer blood, found that *Staphylococcus aureus*-induced B cell proliferation was not significantly affected after an incubation of 1 h at 42 °C in vitro. Jampel et al. (1983) carefully teased out the respective in vitro responses of murine lymphocyte subtypes to 39 °C hyperthermia and concluded that the B cell response to lipopolysaccharide was reduced. Where overall mixed spleen cell lymphocyte proliferation appeared to increase, the hyperthermia-augmented primary humoral response reflected increased helper T cell activity which outweighed any negative effects on B cell function. When murine B cell lymphocytes were heated for 30 min at 42 °C in a water bath by Sulton et al. (1984), B cell "capping" (a function possibly involving B cell differentiation) by antigen-antibody complexes was reduced from 90% to around 10%. The study of Sulton et al. (1984) suggested that the cell membrane is functionally or structurally altered by hyperthermia, especially in the 40 °– 42 °C range. Certainly, scanning electron microscopy reveals changes in lymphocyte surface topology after exposure to hyperthermia (Lin et al. 1973). Roszkowski et al. (1979) found inhibition of membrane ion transport in murine lymphocytes at both 40 ° and 43 °C with incubations ranging from 30 min to 4 h. These membrane changes are probably not specific for B cells; indeed, Kwok et al. (1978) showed a reduction in sodium-dependent amino acid membrane transport in the MOLT4 human T lymphocyte, suggesting impaired protein synthesis. This finding has been used by some to support the argument that the impaired blastogenic response of heated lymphocytes is due to a reduction in the synthesis of proteins required for blastogenesis (Skeen et al. 1983). In a study of another facet of lymphocyte membrane activity, Brewer et al. (1983) reported that following in vitro heating for 1 h at 45 °C, human lymphocytes do not stimulate proliferation of allogeneic lymphocytes in mixed lymphocyte culture (MLC), yet the expression of human leukocyte antigen (HLA)-DR is unchanged and alloantisera to B cell alloantigens are able to recognize HLA-DR determinants on heated cells. This, of course, suggests that simple expression of HLA-DR does not, in itself, indicate stimulation in MLC.

The response of T cells to hyperthermia is probably temperature dependent like most other lymphoid cells, and the differences in results from the various studies reflect hyperthermia dose and differing assay systems. Jampel and his coworkers (1983), using

murine spleen cells in a plaque-forming assay, found that incubation at 39 °C stimulated an antigen-specific immune response. By manipulating lymphocyte subsets independently, they concluded that the helper T cells, or cells generating helper T cells, were preferentially being stimulated. Interestingly, incubation at 39 °C for 15 min was sufficient to induce heat shock proteins in these activated T lymphocytes and they speculated that heat shock proteins might have a role in T cell function.
Mullbacher (1984) studied the antiviral activity of heated lymphocytes. His group demonstrated increased generation of murine secondary influenza virus immune cytotoxic cells in vitro after an 8 h incubation of 39 °C. The maximum activity occurred after 3 – 5 days of culture and suggested to the authors that hyperthermia had accelerated the rate of generation of effector cells.
A number of workers, including Ashman and Nahmias (1977), have found that incubation of human lymphocytes with mitogenic substances such as PHA or concanavalin A (ConA) at elevated temperatures can result in increased incorporation of ^{3}H-thymidine. The results of Ashman and Nahmias, in experiments performed at 39 °C, can be interpreted as showing that either hyperthermia stimulates more cells to produce DNA or simply that hyperthermia increases the rate of DNA synthesis. Hanson et al. (1983) noted that small increases in temperature between 32 ° and 39 °C enhanced ^{3}H-thymidine uptake by thymocytes incubated in the presence of PHA or interleukin-1 (IL-1). The interaction of hyperthermia and cytokines such as IL-1 is discussed in the next section. As incubation temperatures increase above 40 °C however, some workers have shown that transformation responses to mitogens and, in some cases, cell viability appear to decrease (Roberts and Steigbigel 1977).
Furthermore, Roberts et al. (1985) have been able to demonstrate that at temperatures >42.5 °C, DNA, ribonucleic acid (RNA), and total protein synthesis in response to stimulation with optimal concentrations of mitogen is both delayed and reduced.
The foregoing discussion implies that, overall, elevated temperatures in nonphysiological in vitro culture systems may increase T cell function and decrease B cell activity, ignoring any interactive effects with other immune cells. The issue is not clear cut, however. For example, Kalland and Dahlquist (1983) found that at 42 °C, for 1 h, the proliferative response to alloantigens in MLC as well as the T cell mitogen ConA was unaffected. In addition, they noted that the generation of cytotoxic T lymphocytes (CTL) in MLC was unaffected by exposure to heat prior to culture although heat markedly impaired the function of differentiated CTL, suggesting that the degree of differentiation of various lymphoid cell populations may influence their heat sensitivities.

2.2.1 Macrophages and Hyperthermia

Dickson and Shah (1982) have reviewed the studies of Muckle and Dickson who had demonstrated significant macrophage activity accompanying regression of the VX2 carcinoma in the rabbit after hyperthermia. They described further work in rats which suggested that silica-induced depletion of macrophages reduced the effectiveness of hyperthermia in producing cure of tumor-bearing animals.
Stimulation of macrophage activity by *Corynebacterium parvum* injection i.v. (but not i.p.) increased the effectiveness of local hyperthermia against the MC7 sarcoma. This work reinforces the concept of a nonspecific antitumor immunological augmentation in tumor-bearing animals. However, these studies have focused largely on immunogenic tumors. Secondly, in these models, hyperthermia, per se, may have had no direct effect on macrophage function or number but simply induced tumor necrosis, the latter possibly acting as an immunostimulant.

2.2.2 Hyperthermia and NK Cells

Perhaps of greater relevance to the study of neoplasia is the effect of hyperthermia on NK cells. NK cells are a subset of lymphocytes which are able to kill virus-infected cells and tumor cells without prior sensitization (Refs. 1 – 6 in Azocar et al. 1982). They show no major histocompatibility complex restriction for the cytotoxic effect (Zarling and Kung 1980). Several in vivo studies have suggested that reduced or absent NK activity enhances tumor development while NK stimulation achieves the converse (Habu et al. 1981; Hanna 1982). In addition, the NK-deficient mutant beige mouse has increased susceptibility to transplanted tumors (Karre et al. 1980). There appears to be general agreement that at temperatures above 39 °C, NK activity in vitro is reduced (Dinarello et al. 1986). Overall, NK cells appear to be preferentially sensitive to hyperthermia, compared with T or B cells (Kalland and Dahlquist 1983). Studies attempting to restore NK activity following hyperthermia by incubation with cytokines such as interferons at 37 °C have had mixed results (Azocar et al. 1982; Dinarello et al. 1986; Kalland and Dahlquist 1983). Kalland and Dahlquist (1983) showed that hyperthermia interfered both with target cell binding as well as the lytic cycle.

They could not rescue NK activity after 42 °C hyperthermia by incubation overnight with alpha-interferon. Similarly, activation in MLC was also unsuccessful suggesting that pre-NK cells were also heat sensitive.

Azocar et al. (1982) noted similar decreases in NK activity at 40 °C but the reduction was partially offset by the addition of human leukocyte interferon. Dinarello et al. (1986) incubated human lymphocytes at 39 °C for 18 h and noted a similar reduction in NK activity. The addition of IL-1, IL-2, and interferon during the incubation had only a modest effect on abrogating the deleterious effect of hyperthermia. In contrast, Nurmi et al. (1982) were able to restore NK activity following in vitro hyperthermia at 40 °C by exposing them to human leukocyte interferon.

Onsrud (1983) exposed lymphocytes from healthy donors to temperatures ranging from 37 °–42 °C for 1–3 h and then assayed for NK activity. NK effector cells exposed to 42 °C for 1 h lost 90% of their cytotoxic capacity: overnight incubation with interferon at 37 °C did *not* restore activity. There was no significant reduction in cell viability as assessed by trypan blue dye exclusion test. Onsrud noted little effect on T and B cell activity and concluded like Kalland and Dahlquist and others that NK cells are preferentially sensitive to hyperthermia. Kalland and Dahlquist (1983) have suggested that hyperthermic inhibition of NK activity may well be the result of cell membrane damage as has been alluded to by others. Damage to the cell membrane would inhibit recognition of target cells or the processing for lysis.

2.2.3 In Vitro Hyperthermia and Biological Response Modifiers

Several investigators have shown that the pyrogen IL-1 stimulates T cell function and that these effects are enhanced at elevated temperatures (Hanson et al. 1983; Duff and Durum 1982). Duff and Durum (1982) reported that at 39 °C, murine T cell proliferation by IL-1 and IL-2 was significantly enhanced. These workers emphasized the functional interaction of the pyrogenicity and T cell mitogenicity of IL-1 at a temperature consistent with naturally induced fever in the mouse. In contrast, Dinarello et al. (1986) demonstrated that while cytotoxic T cell activity was increased at 39 °C, the production of IL-1, IL-2, erythroid burst-promoting activity, and granulocyte-macrophage colony-stimulating factor by human mononuclear cells was lower at 39 °C than at 37 °C. Taken together, the studies by Duff and Durum (1982) and Dinarello et al. (1986) would suggest that, at temperatures consistent with endogenous pyrexia, certain T cell functions may be enhanced either directly or through increased activity of basal levels of cytokines. However, in vitro production of cytokines and cytokine-primed NK activity appears to be inhibited at 39 °C. It is not clear from the literature what the effect of temperatures higher than 39 °C would be on these functions.

The monokine tumor necrosis factor (TNF) plays an important role in monocyte-macrophage tumor cytotoxicity (Philip and Epstein 1986). It appears that the cytotoxic effects of TNF are enhanced in the 40 °–42 °C temperature range – and this has been established both in vitro and in vivo (Niitsu et al. 1988). The interaction is not simple, however. Klostergaard et al. (1989) have clearly shown that scheduling of the hyperthermia and the monocyte-TNF-triggering lipopolysaccharide is critical. Simultaneous heating (42 °–43 °C) and triggering severely ablated TNF production, whereas lipopolysaccharide administration 90 min prior to heating resulted in enhanced TNF production. Their work suggests that appropriately constructed sequences for either macrophage triggering or monokine treatment of tumor cells combined with hyperthermia could usefully augment the cytotoxic actions of monocytes or macrophages and the cytotoxicity of endogenously added monokines.

Like the interleukins, the interferon cytokines are pyrogenic (Dinarello et al. 1984). Girard et al. (1982) have shown that at 39 °C, mononuclear cell interferon production is decreased. Despite this finding, a series of preclinical investigations has suggested that elevated temperature may potentiate the biological effects of various interferons. Thermal enhancement of the antiproliferative effects of interferon has been demonstrated with Daudi and rat osteosarcoma cells (Delbruck et al. 1980). This enhancement occurred with both partially purified, naturally produced interferon, and interferon produced by recombinant DNA technology purified to homogeneity. A supraadditive antiproliferative effect has also been demonstrated between hyperthermia at 39.5 °C and alpha-interferon in human bladder carcinoma cell lines (Groveman et al. 1984). In these studies, cell lines with a range of sensitivities to interferon were examined; in each case the antiproliferative activity was increased at the elevated temperature. This effect was also correlated with induction of 2, 5-oligoadenylate synthetase, known to be an interferon-inducible enzyme (Merritt et al. 1985). In vivo studies reported by Robins (1984) have also suggested a supraadditive effect of hyperthermia and interferons leading to the development of clinical multimodality WBH studies (Robins et al. 1986c).

2.3 In Vivo Studies: The Abscopal Response and Metastasis

The results of in vivo studies of hyperthermia immunobiology are more controversial than any of the findings of in vitro studies. In many animal tumor models a clear difference has emerged between the apparent immunological sequelae of heating locally and applying some form of WBH (Shah and Dickson 1978a, b). The use of immunogenic transplantable animal tumors and in some cases the high incidence of acute mortality of the WBH subjects make interpretation of the data somewhat difficult. The weight of published opinion, however, has supported an immune-enhancing effect of local hyperthermia in these animal models, whereas WBH has been branded as immunosuppressive (Shah and Dickson 1978a, b).

As outlined in Table 1 there are many unanswered questions about the relevance of measuring either the numbers or activation of individual immune effector cells in vitro following in vivo heating.

Strauss (1969) were the first group to suggest that circulating immunological mediators might be involved in the response of animal tumors to local hyperthermia. They observed regression of tumor at anatomic sites distant from the locally heated primary. Goldenberg and Langner (1971) subsequently observed a similar phenomenon when local hyperthermia treatment of human colon cancer cells implanted in a hamster cheek pouch resulted in regression of tumor in the contralateral cheek pouch. They termed this response to hyperthermia an "abscopal" response, using the word coined by Mole in 1953. In contrast to Goldenberg and Langner, Strauss's group had used a rabbit model. After electrocoagulation of the Brown-Pearce carcinoma growing in the testes of rabbits, regression of the primary tumor and tumor metastases was accompanied by an inconsistent rise in antibody titres in the 2–3 weeks after heating, and this elevated level was maintained for a further 3–4 weeks. Rabbits cured of the disease appeared to be immune to challenge with Brown-Pearce carcinoma cells. Immune sera resulted in tumor regression and host cure when injected into other tumor bearing animals. Unfortunately, the lack of adequate controls, the absence of a detailed description of the methodology employed and the use of a tumor model where spontaneous regression frequently occurs are criticisms which have rendered this work difficult to evaluate.

In better controlled experiments, Shah and Dickson (1978a) studied the effect of local hyperthermia (47 °C for 30 min) on the immune status of rabbits bearing the VX2 carcinoma. Disappearance of both the primary tumor in the leg and distant metastases was accompanied by evidence of augmented humoral and cellular immune response against tumor cells, including a significant macrophage response. It should be noted, of course, that the VX2 carcinoma is an immunogenic tumor. Dickson and Muckle (1972) compared local hyperthermia and WBH using the same animal tumor model, attempting to maintain a tumor temperature at around 42.6 °C for up to 3 h. They demonstrated more rapid tumor destruction after local hyperthermia with half of the animals alive 2 years after hyperthermia, while 13 out of 14 rabbits given WBH were dead with metastatic disease within 1 year. Using the immunological criteria described above, Dickson and Muckle suggested that systemic hyperthermia suppressed or abrogated the immunostimulation induced by heat-damaged tumor cells. Inadequate heating of tumor or stimulation of metastases (see below) by total body heating were alternative explanations offered by these authors. Consistent with the concept of heat-damaged tumor cells acting as an antigenic stimulus are the results of in vitro work by Mondovi et al. (1972) with Ehrlich ascites cells and the work of Tompkins et al. (1981) who treated HCT-8R human tumor cells with hyperthermia for 60 min at 37°–44 °C. Heated cells were sensitized to the cytotoxic action of specific antibodies and complement although there was no increase in antibody binding.

Despite the apparent specificity of the immunological reaction described in the in vitro studies by Tompkins et al., most in vivo studies using a variety of animal tumor models have provided evidence of a rather nonspecific host reaction in response to hyperthermia. Both T and B lymphocytes and macrophages appear to be involved (Dickson and Shah 1982). Urano et al. (1983) have shown in a mouse model that the enhancement of the thermal responses of several types of fibrosarcoma by intravenous injections of *Corynebacterium parvum* was more pronounced for the immunogenic tumors; however, for spontaneous tumors immunogenicity is really demonstrable (Moore 1978). Further evidence for human tumor-associated antigens has been derived solely from in vitro assays and difficulty exists in making correlations with tumor cell kill in vivo (Primm and Baldsin 1978). Thus in man, the evidence for a host immune response after tumor heating is limited.

2.3.1 NK Cells in Vivo

Several groups have attempted to pursue the effect of hyperthermia on NK cell activity in the in vivo situation. Yang et al. (1983) exposed hamsters to a variety of schedules of microwave radiation. A single 24 mW/cm^2, 60-min treatment resulted in a transient depression of splenic NK activity between 4 and 8 h after treatment. This particular microwave radiation technique resulted in a peak core body temperature of 40 °C which was reached in 15 – 30 min. Temperatures returned to normal within about 1 h. Since the reduction in NK activity occurred long after body temperature had returned to normal the authors postulated that a direct effect of hyperthermia on NK cells was unlikely. They were able to correlate the fall and subsequent restoration of NK activity with measured levels of glucocorticosteroids but their own in vitro results of the effects of steroids on NK activity do not wholly support the hypothesis that microwave-induced steroid elevations suppress NK activity in vivo.

Reduced splenic NK activity was also reported by Johnston et al. (1986). His group applied 1 MHz ultrasound (1 – 5 W/cm^2 for 500 s) to the splenic area of anesthetized hamsters. A significant reduction in NK activity was observed 4 h after splenic ultrasound irradiation with a return to control levels by 24 h after treatment. A generalized lymphopenia was noted with a similar time course. Sham-treated animals behaved as controls suggesting that the reduced NK activity was not simply a stress phenomenon.

Rather different effects on NK activity were obtained by Shen et al. (1987). They treated unrestrained, unanesthetized mice bearing either Lewis lung carcinoma of B16 melanoma tumors with 2450-MHz microwave WBH achieving a core temperature of 39.5 °– 40 °C for 30 min 3 or 6 times weekly. They observed an increase in NK activity in tumor-bearing mice and little or no change in normal mice. Of interest, they were able to demonstrate reduced pulmonary metastases in the WBH-treated animals. They confirmed these results in a subsequent study using a different WBH schedule and mice infected with Friend virus complex (Shen et al. 1988).

2.3.2 Metastasis and Hyperthermia

The studies of Shen et al. (1987) highlight one of the more contentious issues concerning the immunological effects of hyperthermia. One of the major controversies in the hyperthermia immunobiology literature has been the issue of promotion or inhibition of tumor metastasis by hyperthermia. Metastasis of cancer cells is a complex phenomenon comprising a sequence of at least five processes (Fidler 1978). The role of hyperthermia in modulating any of these processes is at present not completely understood. The contradictory results in the literature of the effect of either local or WBH on tumor metastasis appear more to reflect the techniques of heating and the assay systems used for measuring metastases than any unifying hypothesis which could pull these varying studies together. For example, it is difficult to interpret the results of Dickson and Ellis (1974) who found that at 1 h, 42 °C water bath heating of the legs of rats bearing the Yoshida sarcoma resulted in increased metastatic spread via lymphatic and vascular routes. The initial experimental results published from this study showed a 90% mortality in the animals so treated and, indeed, this local hyperthermia treatment produced a significant rise in the core temperature, in other words, it resulted in WBH. Since the tumors showed no microscopic evidence of cell necrosis the authors concluded that the enhanced dissemination was due to inadequate heating. In other studies where local hyperthermia has been employed and the measured core temperature has not risen, or risen only negligibly, increased tumor metastasis has not been observed (Ando et al. 1987). In this regard, Yerushalmi (1976) has argued that there needs to be a "gradient" of temperatures between the heated tumor and the rest of the body, i.e., if core temperature rises close to that of the heated tumor, increased metastases will occur.

The data from studies involving WBH and its relation to the promotion or inhibition of tumor metastasis in animals are even more confusing to interpret. Many different heating modalities have been employed including water bath (Oda et al. 1985), hot air (Yerushalmi 1976), incubator (Shah and Dickson 1978a, b), and microwave (Shen et al. 1987). Different WBH temperatures and heating times in different studies compound the difficulty in making comparisons. Several groups, however, appear to have demonstrated an increased number of pulmonary metastases when core temperatures in excess of 41.5° C have been used (Dickson and Muckle 1972; Dickson and Ellis 1974; Yerushalmi 1976; Urano et al. 1983; Oda 1983). Yerushalmi (1976), using hot air incubator, heated mice with Lewis lung tumor implanted in their legs at temperatures of 40.5°– 41.9° C for 10 – 20 min. He purported to show an increase in lung metastases in the animals in whom an elevation of core temperature was obtained. The data was not subjected to statistical scrutiny, however, and the differences between the heated and control animals bearing established tumors as opposed to those treated immediately after tumor cell inoculation were far less convincing. In addition, other workers have shown that the ability of cells to produce tumors after inoculation, certainly for the Walker 256 carcinoma cell line, can be either increased or decreased depending on the WBH heating schedule employed (Brett and Schloerb 1962).

In work referred to earlier, Dickson and Muckle (1972), made a comparison of local hyperthermia versus WBH at a temperature of 42.6° C using the VX2 carcinoma in the rabbit. These authors demonstrated with this immunogenic tumor that not only was whole body heating less effective in controlling the primary tumor, but that there were more metastases in rabbits undergoing WBH. Based on other work published by these authors on the effects of hyperthermia on the immune system of rabbits, Dickson and Muckle postulated that immunosuppression by WBH might be responsible for the increased metastases in the WBH-treated animals. In support of this finding are the results of Doan et al. (1937), and Williams and Galt (1978), who demonstrated lymphoid tissue degeneration in rabbits and rats respectively following WBH at 41° C for varying periods of time.

Lord et al. (1981) reported increased bone metastases after WBH was given to dogs with spontaneous osteosarcoma; however, the metastatic sites were unusual, i.e., bone rather than lung, and no control animals were studied. It is difficult to conclude whether the hyperthermia was directly affecting the pattern of metastasis or whether in fact perhaps the survival time of the animals had increased, allowing for an alteration in the national history of the disease.

Finally it should be noted that one group whose work on NK cells was described earlier, has in fact shown significantly reduced numbers of pulmonary metastases in WBH-treated animals (Shen et al. 1987). The fact that these workers had used an animal tumor model in which contradictory results had been reported by others suggests that many of the conflicting findings reported in the literature may reflect an artifact of the methodology and animal models being employed. Two final points should perhaps be made in regard to the effect of hyperthermia on the phenomenon of metastasis. Firstly, while the predominant speculation has revolved around hyperthermia-induced perturbations of the immune system, other explanations such as heat-induced hyperdynamic circulation have also been invoked (Dickson and Ellis 1974). In addition it should be noted that the presence or absence of local tumor control may not correlate with the frequency of metastasis in WBH-treated animals (Shen et al. 1987).

Laboratory investigations of Neville and Sauder (1988) suggest that WBH (at 41.5°–42° C) and IL-1 may be involved in the metastatic process and that there may be an interaction between them. Using complementary DNA (cDNA) probe for IL-1, these workers measured consistently elevated levels of messenger RNA for IL-1 in the skin of mice undergoing a 1-h, radiant heat, WBH treatment at 41°–42° C. Peak levels were detected at 16–24 h after WBH but levels remained elevated above baseline for 4 days. IL-1 is produced by many types of cells including macrophages, lymphoid, and endothelial cells (Dinarello et al. 1984). The endothelial cell plays a major role in the development of tumor cell metastasis (Adamson et al. 1987). We have hypothesized that 41°–42° C WBH may induce endothelial cell production of IL-1, resulting in increased endothelial adhesiveness for and retention of circulating tumor cells with concomitant increased metastasis development. Preliminary unpublished data show small but significant increases in both lung trapping and subsequent development of pulmonary metastasis in C57B6 mice injected with B16 melanoma cells following IL-1 treatment. WBH alone produced a nonsignificant increase in metastases but increased the effect of IL-1 on the development of metastases.

These in vivo results however, may not simulate the clinical phenomenon of metastasis in established human cancers and there is no evidence as yet that WBH increases the development of metastatic disease in human subjects so treated.

2.4 Clinical Hyperthermia and the Abscopal Response

There are several clinical studies which suggest an abscopal response following clinical hyperthermia. A number of clinical studies have been published on observations using regional hyperthermic limb perfusion in both sarcoma and melanoma (Moricca et al. 1977; Stehlin et al. 1975). The latter workers obtained successful regression of recurrent melanomas of the limbs by regional perfusion with melphalan at 38.8°–40° C. Five-year survival of patients with recurrent cutaneous disease was increased from 22% to 77%. An unspecified number of Stehlin's patients appeared to show an increased "plasma" immunological reaction against their own melanoma cells cultured in vitro, but it is not clear what the authors meant by tumor cell inhibition and no evidence was adduced to support a specific immunological response against melanoma cells. In addition, these were uncontrolled nonrandomized studies. Although the clinical responses were impressive and other workers also subscribe to the position that breakdown products from heated tumor cells act as immunostimulants (Cavaliere et al. 1967), the evidence remains circumstantial. Contradictory evidence has been presented by

Dickson (1984), who treated 11 patients with a variety of extensive recurrent cancers on the chest wall and/or with recurrent deep-seated tumors, with microwave or radio frequency local hyperthermia and irradiation. Hyperthermia was given 4 h after radiation. Dickson found that not only was there little correlation between local tumor regression and overall disease control, but there was no evidence whatsoever of an abscopal response taking place in distant metastatic sites. This issue, therefore, remains unresolved in local-regional hyperthermia and is probably not relevant to WBH.

2.5 Clinical WBH and the Immune Response

As might be expected from perusal of the in vitro and in vivo studies described earlier, an analysis of changes in the immune function of either healthy individuals or cancer patients exposed to an elevated core temperature reveals that the heterogeneity of methodologies and temperatures employed has resulted in a series of inconsistent biological responses (Table 2).

Several complicating factors can be identified in this analysis (see Table 1). Firstly, the identification of a clinically relevant immune parameter to study is difficult given the complex interrelationship of various immune pathways and our lack of understanding of their involvement in the process of human malignancy. Secondly, if such pathways are already disturbed in a patient with an ongoing malignancy, further perturbations as a result of WBH may or may not have any clinical relevance. Thirdly, nearly all WBH methodologies involve some form of sedation or general anesthesia. The latter has been shown to decrease T lymphocyte responses to PHA and bacterial antigens in association with a diminished number of T cells (Berenbaum et al. 1973; Slade et al. 1975). Skin test reactivity is also depressed (Slade et al. 1975). Vose

Table 2. Immunological functions and WBH

Author	Technique	Temperature	Patients	Immune functions
De Horatius et al. (1977)	Water mattress	42 °C	3	WBC ↑; T and B cells, no change in numbers; C3 ↓; antibody-dependent lymphocyte cytotoxicity ↓
Bork-Wolwer et al. (1978)	Water bath	38.5 °C	12 volunteers	T cell fraction of lymphocytes ↓
Gee et al. (1978)	Water bath	41.8 °C	19	T cells, C3, PHA response, antibody-dependent lymphocyte cytotoxicity all ↓. Recovery in 4 days
Parks et al. (1978)	Extracorporeal	42 °C	Numbers not stated	T cells and PHA response ↑; neutrophil cytotoxicity ↑
Fabricius et al. (1978)	Siemens box	40 °C	Volunteers	T cells ↓, PHA response inconsistent
Grogan et al. (1980)	Extracorporeal	41.5° – 42 °C	Numbers not stated	Post-WBH, polymorph, leukocyte bactericidal activity ↑ (tested at 37 °C). In vitro at 42 °C, polymorph, leukocyte bactericidal activity ↓
Zanker and Lange (1982)	Extracorporeal	41.8 °C	1	NK cells ↑
Koga et al. (1983)	Extracorporeal	41.5° – 42 °C	8	PHA response ↓; skin reaction to PPD and PHA ↓; rosetting ↓; C3 ↓; IgG ↓. Recovery after 1 week
Wiedmeyer et al. (1983)	Radiant heat	41.8 °C	3	1 h after peak temp., response to soluble antigens ↓; 1 week after WBH, normal response
Downing and Taylor (1987)	Water bath	39 °C	Numbers not stated	NK cells ↑; T (helper) ↓; TNF, no change; IL-2 production ↑

PHA, phytohemagglutinin; *PPD*, purified protein derivative and Moudgil (1976) reported a postoperative reduction in antibody-dependent lymphocyte-mediated cytotoxicity following anesthesia.

One of the first studies of immune changes in cancer patients undergoing WBH was published by De Horatius et al. (1977). They examined three patients, two of whom also received chemotherapy. While rapid rosetting (a measure of T cell activity) did rise acutely following WBH (42° C, 2 h), overall T cell and B cell numbers changed little and antibody-dependent lymphocyte cytotoxicity was depressed. The time course of the changes in immune activity assessed by these authors was not described.

Several of the studies in Table 2 have addressed the issue of the time course of the hyperthermic perturbations in immune function (Gee et al. 1978; Koga et al. 1983). While many groups have reported reduced immunological function following WBH, the changes, even if significant, appear transient. One interesting case report from Zanker and Lange (1982) describes the time course of changes in NK cell activity in a 17-year-old boy with metastatic Ewing sarcoma resistant to chemotherapy and radiation. Two hours after a 6-h 41.8° C WBH treatment (extracorporeal technique) peripheral blood lymphocytes exhibited an NK activity of 30% compared to nearly zero prior to treatment. This elevation lasted for about 7 days at which time the level dropped to 10%. Four days after a second similar WBH treatment, NK activity rose to over 60%. This report, of course, remains anecdotal but elevations in NK activity following "mild" hyperthermic increases in core temperature to 39° C were noted in normal volunteers heated in a water bath by Downing and Taylor (1987). As in most of these studies the immunoassays were performed at 37° C. In their 1987 publication, Downing and Taylor alluded to previous work from their group which demonstrated that, in both the rhesus monkey and man, WBH enhances the subsequent synthesis of gamma interferon in mitogen-stimulated mononuclear cell cultures. They then reported that while IL-2 production and NK activity increased at an unspecified time after WBH, lipopolysaccharide-induced TNF synthesis in monocyte cultures was unchanged and lymphocyte transformation responses to mitogens were actually depressed. Thus, depending on which parameter was chosen as important, one could argue that the hyperthermia was immunosuppressive, immunostimulatory, or had no effect.

As a postscript to this discussion of the effects of clinical WBH on the immune system, one clinical observation made by several workers in this field is perhaps worth describing. Pettigrew et al. (1974b) in their original paper noted that 20%–40% of their patients developed circumoral herpes simplex lesions following their initial treatment. Similar findings were noted by Bull et al. (1979b), Barlogie et al. (1979), and Larkin et al. (1977). This observation, which is common enough in interferon-treated patients, may simply be an epiphenomenon of WBH treatment and one can speculate as to whether it represents nothing more than a transient alteration of antiviral immunity.

What can the clinician interested in hyperthermia glean from this miscellany of reports of immune changes during WBH? The clinical evidence presented thus far does not allow for either exaggerated optimism that WBH can be usefully combined with immunotherapy, nor undue pessimism that the observed changes in immune function would necessarily detract from the potential therapeutic benefit of the WBH itself. Extrapolating from in vitro and in vivo studies of interferon activity at elevated temperatures (described earlier), Robins et al. (1986c) have performed a phase I study of WBH in conjunction with human lymphoblastoid interferon (IFN-α Ly) in 17 patients with advanced cancer.

Table 3. Effect of therapy on BRM parameters after WBH and IFN

BRM assay	Treatment		
	WBH alone pretreatment vs 24 h after pretreatment	IFN alone pretreatment vs day 6	IFN-WBH pretreatment vs day 6
2-5A synthetase	2% ↓ ($p = 0.92$)	500% ↑ ($p < 0.0001$)	470% ↑ ($p < 0.0001$)
β_2-microglobulin	5% ↓ ($p = 0.30$)	92% ↑ ($p < 0.0001$)	110% ↑ ($p < 0.0001$)
Natural killer	3% ↑ ($p = 0.89$)	65% ↑ ($p = 0.02$)	80% ↑ ($p = 0.09$)
Antibody-dependent cellular toxicity	15% ↑ ($p = 0.54$)	54% ↑ ($p = 0.08$)	110% ↑ ($p = 0.03$)
Serum IFN levels	Not significant ↑	↑ Proportional to IFN given	Not different from IFN alone

BRM, biological response modulation; *2-5A*, 2′5′-oligoadenylate synthetase

The study design incorporated a treatment schedule which allowed comparisons of WBH alone, IFN administered i.m., and combinations of the two modalities. IFN-α Ly was given for 6 days in weeks 2, 4, and 6. At least five patients were entered at each of three IFN dose levels (1×10^6 units/m^2; 3×10^6 units/m^2; 10×10^6 units/m^2). WBH was delivered on day 1 of week 1, day 6 of week 4, and days 4 and 6 of week 6. IFN was administered 1 h prior to WBH. The schedule used allowed for the development of tachyphylaxis to IFN-induced fever. Maximum temperatures were not significantly higher 24 h after IFN-WBH than after a comparable number of days of IFN-α Ly alone. There was no statistically significant difference 24 h after treatment in serum IFN levels, or biological response modulation (i.e., 2′,5′-oligoadenylate synthetase activity; β_2-microglobulin levels; natural killer cell cytotoxicity, using K562 target cells and Chang cells) using either IFN-α Ly alone or combined modality therapy (see Table 3). There was, however, a trend toward greater enhancement of NK cell and antibody-dependent cellular toxicity with the combination of IFN and WBH. Statistically significant validation of such a trend will require further clinical investigations. Based on the results of this clinical study Robins et al. (1986c) concluded that combined modality therapy was well tolerated, with no untoward toxicities. The maximum tolerated dose of IFN-α Ly which was recommended for phase II IFN-WBH trials was 3×10^6 units/m^2. (This trial, which reported clinical responses, was not designed to demonstrate whether WBH improved the therapeutic effect of interferon.) No other clinical studies of a similar nature have as yet been reported.

2.6 Conclusions

Both endogenous fever and exogenously applied hyperthermia appear to exert a number of complex, albeit transient and poorly understood changes on the immune system. For the multitude of reasons described in this review, difficulties remain in extrapolating the results of either in vitro or animal experiments to the clinical WBH situation. Further clinical studies of the immune function of cancer patients undergoing hyperthermia treatments will be necessary before any definitive statement can be made about the significance of any interaction between hyperthermia and elements of the immune system.

3 WBH and Ionizing Irradiation

3.1 Background

Preclinical in vitro and in vivo studies suggest that hyperthermia enhances the sensitivity of tumor cells to ionizing irradiation at temperatures consistent with ~42° C WBH (Belli and Bointi 1963; Ben-Hur and Elkind 1974; Ben-Hur et al. 1972, 1974; Cater et al. 1964; Gerweck et al. 1975; Henle and Leeper 1976; Kim, JH et al. 1974; Overgaard and Overgaard 1972; Robinson and Wizenberg 1974). Conceptually this phenomenon could result from the cumulative effects of at least four distinct processes.

One of these processes might be true radiosensitization – the ability of heat to increase the amount of damage caused by a given dose of irradiation. For example, induction of singe-stranded DNA breaks can be modestly increased by combined heat and irradiation (Corry et al. 1977; Mills and Meyn 1981; Jorritsma and Konings 1984) (evidence of increased induction of double-stranded breaks between 41° and 46° C [Corry et al. 1977] is however lacking). Increased damage could result from changes in the amount and conformation of DNA-associated proteins following heating. These changes correlate with thermal enhancement of radiosensitivity in some experimental systems (Corry et al. 1977; Mills and Meyn 1981, 1983; Roti and Winward 1978; Tomasovic et al. 1978). Conceivably, disrupting the structure or function of nucleoproteins could increase the physical exposure of DNA to irradiation or affect the access of repair enzymes to DNA (Corry et al. 1977). Interpretation of the preceding studies is complicated by the observation that heat itself might induce DNA strand breakage (Corry et al. 1977; Jorritsma and Konings 1984).

A second mechanism might involve thermal inhibition of the repair of sublethal and potentially lethal radiation damage to DNA. There is little doubt that heat exposure at temperatures above 43° C modifies DNA repair after a given irradiation. The rate of repair of single-stranded DNA breaks is significantly slowed down by heat exposure at these temperatures (Bowden and Kusanic 1981; Clark et al. 1981; Corry et al. 1977; Jorritsma et al. 1985; Lunec et al. 1981; Mills and Meyn 1981, 1983; Warters et al. 1987). Several hours after a heat exposure at 43° C (Mills and Meyn 1981) or 45° C (Clark et al. 1981) the rate of single-strand repair returns essentially to normal in conjunction with the resolution of much of the thermal radiosensitization effect.

Such observations should be interpreted in the context of evidence which shows that single-stranded breaks are probably not the radiation injury which ultimately causes cell death (Chadwick and Leenhouts 1973; Dugle et al. 1976; Mills and Meyn 1983). Rather, residual strand breaks which remain after a long period of repair may better account for cytotoxicity (Mills and Meyn 1983; Ritter et al. 1977; Roots et al. 1979). Double-stranded DNA breaks, which can be measured using neutral elution techniques, might constitute a major portion of this residual damage and appear to be responsible for much of the radiation killing (Dugle et al. 1976; Mills and Meyn 1983; Radford 1983; Ritter et al. 1977; Ward 1981).

One study by Mills and Meyn clearly illustrates the potential relationship between heating and decreased repair of residual DNA damage. These investigators found that 43°–45° C hyperthermia before irradiation increases residual DNA breaks (Mills and Meyn 1983). The frequency of residual DNA breaks increased with temperature and with the duration of heating (Mills and Meyn 1983). Significantly, when the sequence of heat and irradiation was varied, the frequency of residual DNA breaks correlated well with the degree of enhancement of radiation killing (Figs. 1 and 2). Radiosensitivity and the levels of residual strand breaks returned to normal when heat and irradiation were separated by 8 h or more (Mills and Meyn 1983); DNA-associated proteins were found to return to normal in about the same time (Mills and Meyn 1983).

When considering the WBH setting, enthusiasm for the "DNA repair" school of thought must be tempered by the observation that the aforementioned studies utilized temperatures above 42.0° C and that most investigators have not detected changes in rates

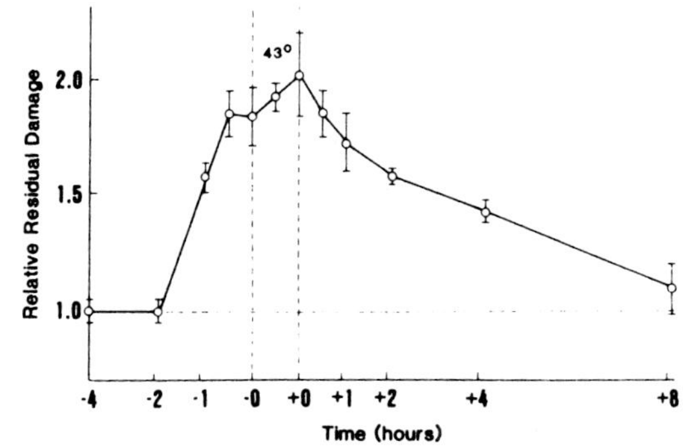

Fig. 1. Effect of varying the sequence of heat and radiation on the relative levels of residual DNA damage. Cells were either irradiated with 5000 rad of 250-kV(p)X-rays or treated for 1 h at 43 °C and then given the alternative treatment at various times afterward. Cells were maintained at 37 °C between the two treatments. In all cases the cells received a total of 8 h of postirradiation incubation at 37 °C. The *two vertical dashed lines* show the time of heat treatment and the *individual points* are plotted to show the time of irradiation in relationship to the heat treatment; the *points to the left* of the vertical dashed lines represent irradiation prior to heat; the *point between the dashed lines*, samples irradiated during the heat treatment; and *points to the right*, cells irradiated after heat. The values shown are relative to a value of 1.0 for cells that received irradiation alone and 8 h of repair. No DNA strand breaks were detected in cells which received heat alone. Each *point* represents the average and standard deviation of three independent determinations (Mills and Meyn 1983)

of DNA repair with heating at or below 42° C even though such an increase is often apparent in the same cell lines at higher temperatures (see Fig. 3).

Furthermore, 41.5° C hyperthermia and irradiation produce clearly supraadditive killing in a human acute lymphoblastic leukemia cell line even though the cell line has very limited DNA repair capabilities (Cohen et al. 1988; Robins et al. 1990a). It should also be noted that 43° C hyperthermia could alter enzyme structure but lower temperatures might predominantly affect enzyme function. It is therefore interesting that 41°–42° C hyperthermia (after irradiation) appears to accelerate the rates of DNA repair in at least three experimental systems (Ben-Hur and Elkind 1974; Dikomey 1982; Warters et al. 1987).

Evidence that WBH might inhibit DNA repair can be derived from the observation by Corry and coworkers that heat-affected repair at temperatures from 41° to 46° C (Corry et al. 1977). Consistent with Corry's studies is the observation that 42° C hyperthermia slows the repair of single-stranded breaks induced in vitro by methylmethane sulfonate, an alkylating agent (Bronk et al. 1973).

Studies of clinical samples obtained from patients undergoing WBH at the University of Wisconsin Clinical Cancer Center (Jonsson et al. 1987) suggest

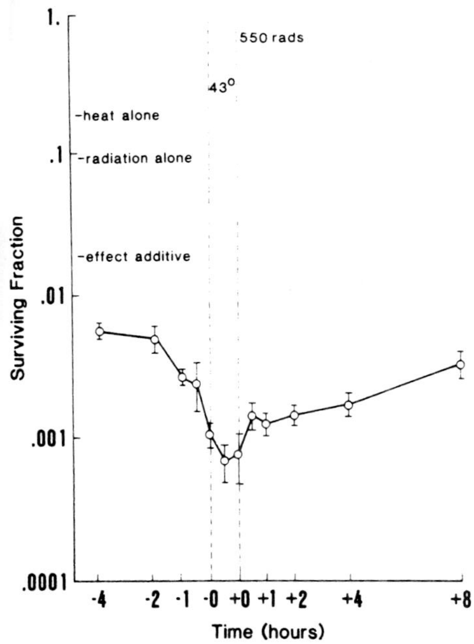

Fig. 2. Effect of varying the sequence of heat and radiation on cell survival. The protocol for this experiment was identical to that described for Fig. 1 except that the end point was cell survival instead of DNA strand breaks and the cells received an X-ray dose of 550 rad. Each *point* represents the average and standard deviation of three independent determinations. The surviving fractions associated with heat alone, radiation alone, and effect additive are indicated (Mills and Meyn 1983)

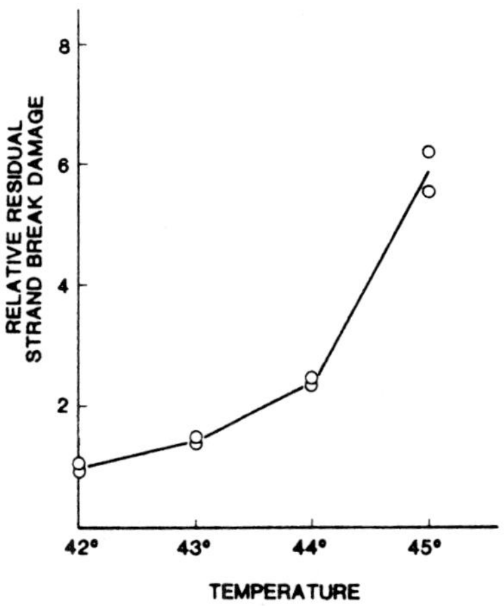

Fig. 3. Relative residual DNA strand-break damage as a function of temperature of a hyperthermia treatment. Cells were treated at various temperatures for 30 min just prior to irradiation with 5000 rad of ^{137}Cs γ-rays. The cells were then incubated for 8 h at 37 °C and the amount of residual unrejoined DNA strand breaks was determined using alkaline elution. The resulting profiles were analyzed in terms of equivalent radiation damage and the relative increase in such damage after the hyperthermia treatments was calculated by dividing the values obtained by the amount of equivalent radiation damage measured in cells that received irradiation alone. No DNA strand breaks were detected in cells that received heat alone. The results from two independent experiments are shown (Mills and Meyn 1983)

a possible mechanism by which WBH could affect DNA repair. The nicotinamide-adenine dinucleotide (NAD) and ATP contents of peripheral lymphocytes were measured just prior to and immediately following WBH treatment of five patients who suffered from various malignancies. The core temperature was 41.8° C for 90–140 min. The levels of both nucleotides decreased by at least 30% in each patient. These effects were duplicated in cultured lymphocytes heated with the same temperature-time profile. The nucleotide depletion was not due to hyperthermia-induced NAD consumption via mono- or poly(ADP ribosylation) reactions or due to leakage through the cell membrane, but was probably due to heat-induced changes in cellular energy metabolism.

The fact that NAD levels decrease following heat treatment could have important implications with regard to treating patients with combinations of hyperthermia and radiation or DNA-damaging drugs. NAD levels in many immature and proliferating cells are lower than in their normal counterparts and near or below the K_m value for poly(ADP ribose) polymerase, an important DNA repair enzyme. Any further decrease in NAD levels may limit DNA repair by this enzyme. Low NAD and ATP pools may also disrupt energy metabolism during the critical period required for appropriate DNA repair.

In addition to the above considerations, a third possible radiosensitization mechanism could be partial cell cycle synchronization by hyperthermia (Kal et al. 1975; Mini et al. 1986; Sapozink et al. 1973) which could then influence radiosensitivity (Li and Kal 1977; Palzer and Heidelberger 1973b; Westra and Dewey 1971). Conversely, irradiation also perturbs the cell cycle distribution of a cell population (e.g., Kal et al. 1975) which could affect thermal sensitivity (Kal et al. 1975; Dewey et al. 1971; Westra and Dewey 1971). Finally, in a fourth possible mechanism, heat can give the appearance of enhancing radiation killing as a consequence of the differential heat and radiation sensitivities of various cell subpopulations. Well oxygenated, proliferating cells with normal pH and adequate nutrition (Fig. 4) are relatively sensitive to irradiation and resistant to hyperthermic killing; poorly oxygenated, nonproliferating cells at low pH in nutritionally restricted microenvironments are radiation resistant but very sensitive to thermal killing (Dewey et al. 1977a, b; Dickson and Oswald 1976; Freeman et al. 1977; Gerweck 1982; Gerweck et al. 1974; Gerweck and Rottinger 1976; Hahn 1974; Hofer and Mivechi 1980; Kim et al. 1975 a, b; Li and Kal 1977; Overgaard 1981b; Sapareto 1978a, b; Suit and Swayder 1974). In addition, heat and irradiation preferentially kill cells in different phases of the cell cycle

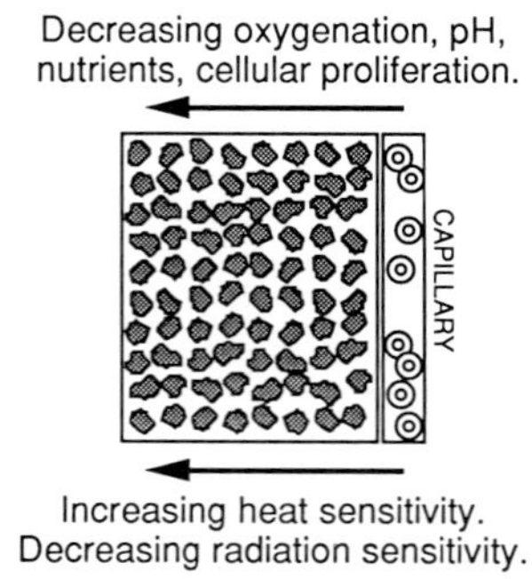

Fig. 4. The relationship between selected microenvironmental factors and cellular sensitivity to heat or irradiation killing

(Harisiadis et al. 1975; Palzer and Heidelberger 1973a; Westra and Dewey 1971).

When we attempt to describe the end result of this potential interaction (i.e., tumor cell death) we must carefully consider our use of terms and the homogeneity of the cell population being studied. To provide such a framework, Fig. 5 gives a functional definition of synergistic, antagonistic, and independent effects with regard to the end point of cell killing in a *homogeneous cell sample* (Dewey 1984).

In this hypothetical example, tumor cell survival after a single exposure to hyperthermia is 50% (Fig. 5b). After a single irradiation, survival also happens to be 50% (Fig. 5c). Survival when both agents are given

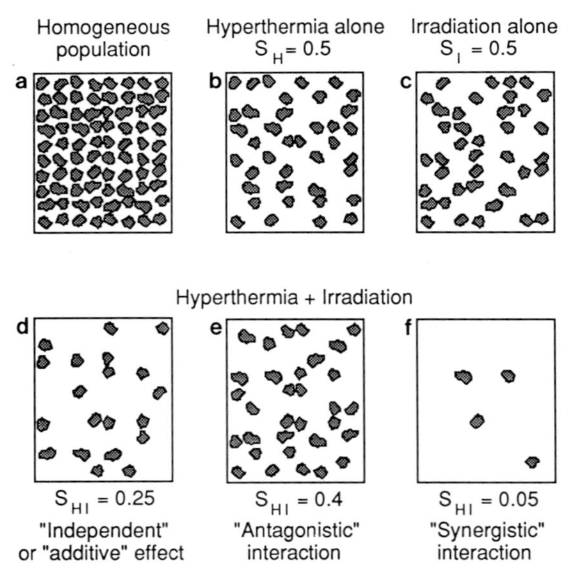

Fig. 5a–f. Effects of a given heat exposure and a given radiation dose in a completely homogeneous cell population (**a**). Heat alone or radiation alone reduces cellular survival to 50% (**b**, **c**). Together, heat and irradiation have independent (**d**), antagonistic (**e**), or synergistic (**f**) cytotoxic interactions. S_H, single exposure to hyperthermia; S_I, single exposure to irradiation; S_{HI}, single exposure to hyperthermia and irradiation

(Fig. 5d–f) can fall into three patterns which *imply* but do not prove three types of interactions. First, the survival after combination therapy might be precisely what would be predicted given the effects of the two modalities as single agents. That is, $0.25 = 0.5 \times 0.5$ or $S_{HI} = S_H \times S_I$, suggesting that hyperthermia and irradiation do not interact (Fig. 5d). Alternatively, the survival after combination therapy might be greater than what was expected. That is, $S_{HI} > S_H \times S_I$ (e.g., $0.4 > 0.5 \times 0.5$ as in Fig. 5e). This implies that hyperthermia and irradiation have antagonistic effects on cell killing. Ideally $S_{HI} < S_H \times S_I$, which we would call synergistic killing (e.g., $0.05 < 0.5 \times 0.5$ as in Fig. 5f). These definitions do not apply to clinical or experimental settings involving *heterogeneous* cell populations. For heterogeneous populations it is more appropriate to use descriptive terms which do not infer the actual mechanisms involved. For example, in the simplified situation of Fig. 6a, hyperthermia is killing 50% of the net tumor cell population but poorly oxygenated cells at lower pH are especially being killed. Irradiation also kills 50% but in this case well-oxygenated, rapidly replicating cells are disproportionately being injured (Fig. 6b).

Figure 6c shows a situation in which heat and irradiation do not appear to interact; they *appear* to have "independent" effects ($S_{HI} = S_H \times S_I$). For comparison, in Fig. 6d, $S_{HI} > S_H \times S_I$, which *implies* an "antagonistic" interaction between the two treatments.

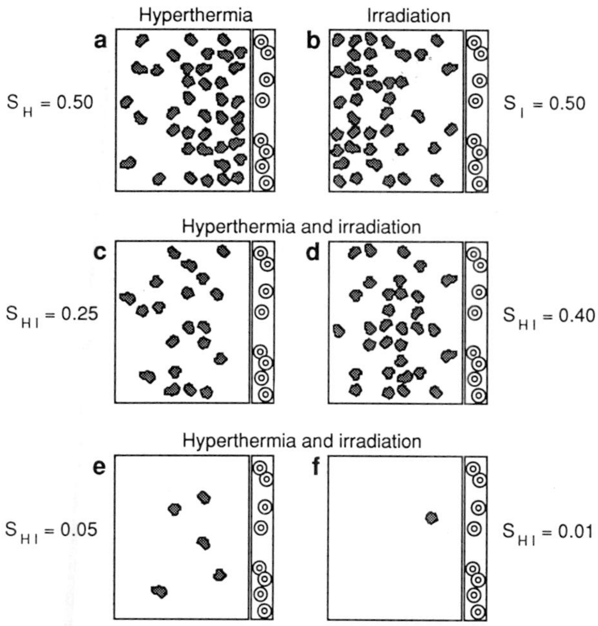

Fig. 6a–f. Potential effects of a given heat exposure and a given radiation dose in a nonhomogeneous population of cells which have variable pH, degrees of oxygenation, or nutritional status. Heat alone or irradiation alone kills 50% of the cells (**a**, **b**). Together, heat and irradiation can have *apparently* independent (**c**), antagonistic (**d**) or supraadditive (**e**, **f**) cytotoxic interactions

Figure 6e and f portray two closely related situations which could correspond very closely to the actual interaction between WBH and irradiation in vivo. Figure 6e shows "supraadditive" killing in that $S_{HI} < S_H \times S_I$. In this case, hyperthermia and irradiation are affecting different tumor cell populations so $S_{HI} < S_H \times S_I$, despite the fact that hyperthermia is not affecting radiosensitivity whatsoever.

In Fig. 6f heat and irradiation preferentially kill different cell populations but heat also increases the sensitivity of all cells to irradiation. The radiosensitizing effect should be greater in hypoxic, acidotic, nutritionally deprived cells as opposed to nutritionally "normal" tumor cells – one effect which explains how hyperthermia theoretically might improve the therapeutic index of irradiation (Gillette and Ensley 1979; Hahn 1974; Hofer and Mivechi 1980; Robinson and Wizenberg 1974; Robinson et al. 1974). In view of this scenario Fig. 6c could actually reflect the presence of a weak antagonistic interaction (i.e., S_{HI} should be less than 0.25 even without thermal radiosensitization).

As we have tried to show, multiple processes could contribute to the cumulative supraadditive toxicity which is observed when hyperthermia and irradiation are combined. Henceforth, for lack of a better descriptive term, we will refer collectively to these multiple phenomena as "thermal radiosensitization" recognizing that a gross oversimplification is thus being imposed.

The efficacy of hyperthermia in enhancing radiation sensitivity can be described by calculating a thermal enhancement ratio (TER). In vivo the most objectively defined end point is usually tumor control (or response) where TCDn is the dose of irradiation which controls tumors in "n" percent of the treated animals. For tumors in vivo the TER can be defined as TCDn (generally TCD50) with radiation only divided by TCDn when both heat and irradiation are given (Fig. 7). In vitro a similar calculation can be made using the survival curves for irradiation alone and for both agents together as is shown in Fig. 8. Generally, WBH temperatures produce TERs (in vitro or in vivo) of at least 1.4–1.7 (e.g., 1.43 and 1.65 [Cohen et al. 1988], 1.6 [Steeves et al. 1987]).

It is frequently assumed that a positive TER will translate into some increase in the therapeutic index for irradiation. This assumption is not necessarily valid as thermal radiosensitization occurs in both neoplastic as well as normal tissue (Gillette and Ensley 1979; Law et al. 1977; Morris et al. 1977; Myers and Field 1977; Robinson et al. 1974; Stewart and

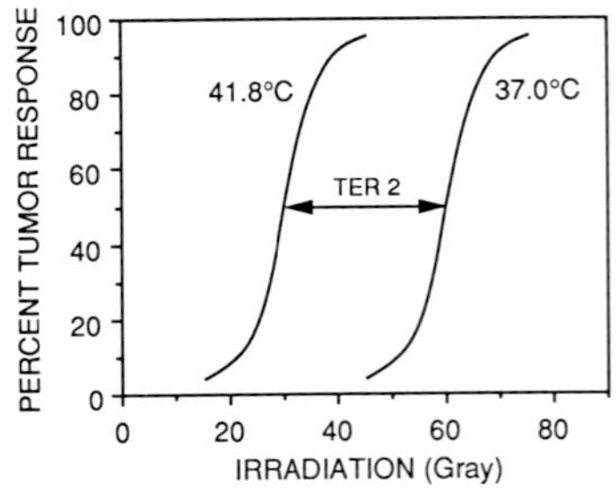

Fig. 7. Relationship between probability of tumor response to irradiation at two temperatures for a hypothetical tumor in vivo. A commonly employed method for describing thermal enhancement ratio (*TER*) is based on a ratio of the doses needed to achieve a given tumor response at the two temperatures

Denekamp 1977; Stewart and Denekamp 1978; Thrall et al. 1975). As a result we must compare the relative effects of heat on both normal and neoplastic tissues. This comparison can be made by calculating a therapeutic gain factor equal to the TER for tumor tissue divided by the TER for normal tissue (e.g., Gillette and Ensley 1979; Robinson et al. 1974).

For the WBH-irradiation setting, the issue of therapeutic index has been partially addressed in one in vivo study by Steeves et al. (1987). These workers concluded that ionizing irradiation and hyperthermia provided supraadditive killing of leukemia cells in the AKR murine model. This positive interaction was more effective in attacking leukemia cells than normal hematopoietic stem cells as was suggested by the longer survival of AKR mice bearing leukemic ascites grafts following TBI and WBH. This selective radiosensitization was further documented by the different survival curves of normal and leukemic cells irradiated and heated in vitro.

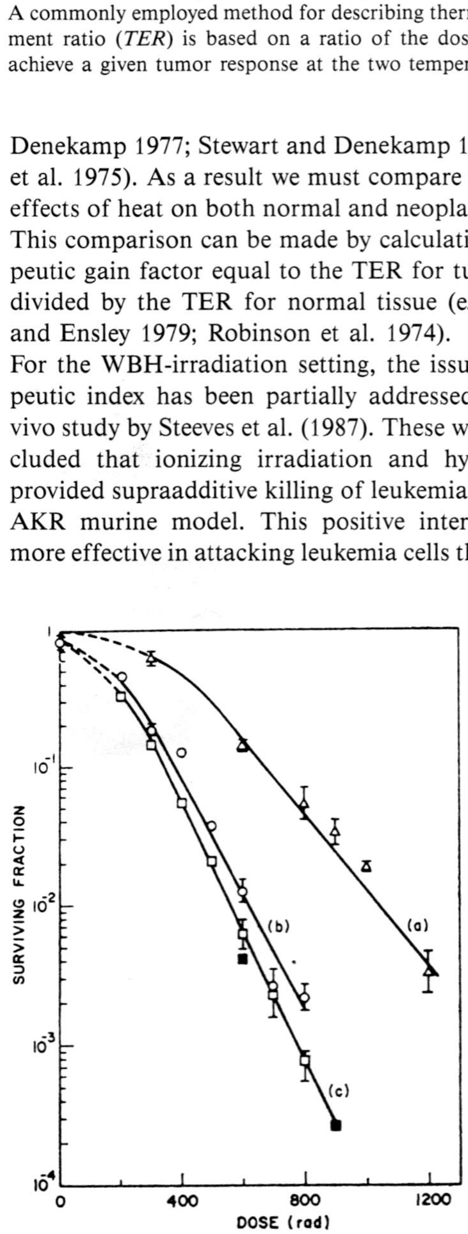

Fig. 8. HA-1 cells in Eagles minimum essential medium (MEM) (with 15% Fetal Bovine Serum) (FBS). (*a*) irradiation alone; (*b*) irradiation plus heat treatment at 43 °C for 60 min; (*c*) heat treatment at 43 °C for 60 min plus irradiation (Li and Kal 1977)

3.2 Potential Advantages of WBH Compared to Local Hyperthermia

It is hoped that systemic hyperthermia will improve the probability of tumor cure or of local tumor control in common radiotherapy situations. In this regard, it should be noted that radiant heat WBH achieves a relatively uniform temperature elevation throughout the body except for limited "partial sanctuary" sites which are slightly cooler as we discuss in Chaps. 5 and 6. This situation is vastly different from the local hyperthermia setting where tissue temperatures vary dramatically even within a given tumor mass as a function of exogenous energy input, tissue blood flow rates, microvascular response, local tissue metabolic rate, and position relative to the energy source (Song 1984).

The marked temperature inhomogeneity of local hyperthermia has important clinical ramifications (Dewhirst et al. 1987) in view of the results of prospective, randomized clinical (Oleson et al. 1984b), and veterinary (Dewhirst and Sim 1984a, b; Dewhirst et al. 1984) studies combining local hyperthermia and irradiation. These studies have observed that the lowest temperature recorded within a tumor is a strong predictor of tumor response. Indeed, the minimum temperature has greater prognostic significance than do the size, histology, location, or radiation dose of a tumor (Dewhirst et al. 1984; Sim et al. 1984). Conversely, the highest recorded temperature correlates strongly with normal tissue damage (Dewhirst and Sim 1984a; Luk et al. 1981).

In this light, the uniformity achieved by WBH is potentially quite valuable since curative radiotherapy strategies for many malignancies (e.g., primary lung neoplasms, Hodgkin's disease, etc.) require irradiation of deeply situated tumor masses or irradiation of large treatment fields. Local hyperthermia, in contrast, is usually limited to the palliation of relatively small and superficial lesions which can be encompassed by existing local hyperthermia devices (Meyer 1984a).

WBH temperatures are also high enough to affect the terminal slope (D_0) and "shoulder" (D_q) of radiation survival curves to a clinically meaningful extent in a

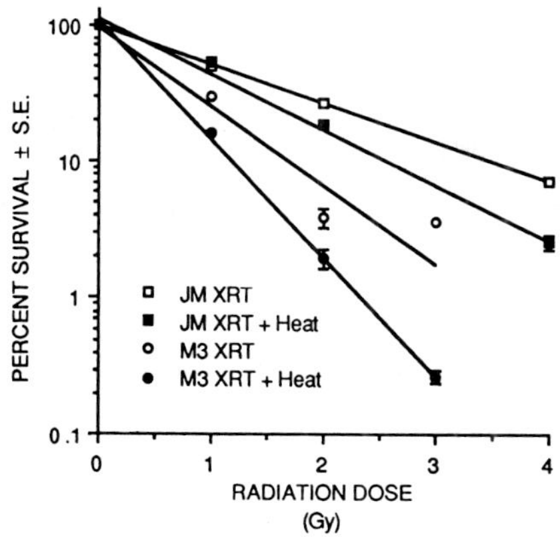

Fig. 9. Sensitivity of JM and MOLT3 cells to irradiation with and without pre-irradiation hyperthermia. Cells received heat treatment for 1 h at 37.0 or 41.5 °C immediately before varying doses of irradiation. Data for combined heat and irradiation are corrected for direct heat killing. *Bars*, SE (Cohen et al. 1988)

variety of human and animal tumors (Cohen et al. 1988; Raaphorst and Azzan 1983; Sapareto et al. 1978a; Steeves et al. 1987). As an example, Fig. 9 shows the effect of 41.5° C hyperthermia (for 1 h) on the radiation survival of JM and MOLT3 cells, two human T cell acute lymphoblastic leukemia cell lines whose radiation survival curves do not display a shoulder effect. For JM and MOLT3 cells the thermal enhancement ratios are 1.43 and 1.65, respectively (Cohen et al. 1988).

3.3 The Importance of Treatment Temperatures Used in Preclinical Studies

Many studies which have profoundly influenced perceptions about thermal radiosensitization have also employed temperatures well above 42° C, with heating at 43°–46° C being used in nearly every reference cited in this chapter. By comparison, only a few studies have addressed thermal radiosensitization at 42° C or cooler (Cohen et al. 1988; Corry et al. 1977; Holahan et al. 1984; Raaphorst et al. 1983; Sapareto et al. 1978a; Steeves et al. 1987).

The frequent decision to study high temperatures might reflect an intended relevance to clinical local hyperthermia where some have expected to reach 43° C or higher (Meyer 1984a). Ironically, most local hyperthermia devices have difficulty in uniformly achieving temperatures higher than 41 °–42 °C except in the very central portions of the treatment region (Aristizabal and Oleson 1984; Meyer 1984a).

We have raised this topic because it is not clear whether experiments involving high temperatures (i.e., >42 °C) are relevant to the systemic hyperthermia setting at or below 41.8 °C (Cohen et al. 1988). Abundant evidence suggests that cells are injured by qualitatively different mechanisms at different temperatures. One hint that this is so is the repeated observation that cells are killed at distinctly different rates at temperatures above and below about 42 °–43 °C. This observation is compatible with the idea that thermal killing is really the cumulative result of multiple types of heat damage, each of which occurs in its own temperature range. Protein denaturation, for example, occurs at 43 °C or higher but is difficult to detect at lower temperatures (Dewey et al. 1977a). Similarly, in one experimental system heat itself caused DNA strand breaks at temperatures above 43 °C but did not detectably do so at lower temperatures (Jorritsma and Konings 1984). Finally, as we have just mentioned, 41 °–42 °C hyperthermia might actually accelerate DNA repair whereas higher temperatures clearly inhibit DNA repair.

An argument could be made as follows: Thermal injury (but not necessarily thermal killing [Mivechi and Hofer 1983]) is a clear prerequisite for the supraadditive cytotoxicity which we are calling thermal radiosensitization (e.g., Sapareto et al. 1978a). Some of this radiosensitization could reflect hyperthermic inactivation of cellular processes that repair radiation damage. Different types of hyperthermic damage occur in different temperature ranges. Therefore, it is conceivable that heat inactivates *qualitatively* different repair mechanisms at different temperatures. Analogous arguments can easily be made regarding the three other potential mechanisms for thermal radiosensitization that were described earlier.

For the reasons we have cited, it is possible that many conclusions in the general thermal radiosensitization literature simply do not apply to radiosensitization in the systemic hyperthermia setting. Unfortunately, it is this general literature that we must use if we are to adequately review radiosensitization by WBH, a broad and potentially complex topic. In so doing we have attempted to locate every thermal radiosensitization study involving temperatures below 42 °C and we have cited only a small fraction of the "higher temperature" literature. Yet, studies focusing predominantly on WBH temperatures comprise only 6 of the 99 references that we are able to cite in this chapter (excluding 3 clinical studies). Hopefully, this situation will improve in the near future. For the present we must cautiously consider the applicability of most data to the special topic of systemic hyperthermia.

3.4 Possibly Controllable Clinical Treatment Variables

Thermal radiosensitization is potentially affected by at least six factors which can be at least partially controlled by the clinician. These are the treatment temperature, the duration of heating, the sequence in which cells are heated and irradiated, the interval between the two modalities ("treatment interval"), the fractionation of treatments, and the phenomenon of thermal tolerance. Theoretically, it should be possible to optimize the tumoricidal efficacy of WBH with irradiation by carefully considering these treatment aspects. A more important consideration is how to optimize the therapeutic index of combination therapy. It should be remembered that a factor which increases cytotoxicity might improve, worsen, or not affect the therapeutic index.

Treatment temperature and heating duration are important considerations to the extent that higher temperatures and longer heating durations cause more severe thermal injury and should result in greater thermal radiosensitization. By this reasoning treatment temperatures should be as high as is safe, i.e., 41.8 °C (Robins et al. 1985b), and the length of systemic hyperthermia should be as long as is clinically practical. This view is reinforced by evidence that 41.5 °C hyperthermia causes greater radiosensitization than does the only slightly lower 41.0 °C in some experimental systems (e.g., Sapareto et al. 1979).

In making such a suggestion we expect to maximize just the end point of thermal radiosensitization. It is expected that other factors (e.g., low pH, hypoxia, etc. as described previously) will provide for the differential radiosensitization of tumor and normal tissues by the combination therapy.

Very little can be said with regard to the ideal duration of WBH as only a few studies have considered this topic (Cohen et al. 1988). One available example, involving two human T cell acute lymphoblastic leukemia cell lines (JM and MOLT3), is shown in Fig. 10. For these cell lines, net killing (heat and irradation) and thermal radiosensitization (measured by survival < 100% after correction for thermal killing) both increase with increasing durations of preirradiation 41.5 °C hyperthermia (although thermal radiosensitization does not appear until heating durations exceed 20 min). For MOLT3 cells it appears that one should certainly heat for at least 3 h. In sharp contrast, for JM cells, 100 min seems best since longer heating adds no further radiosensitization.

Based on these results it is possible to get a very rough feeling of the heating durations necessary to achieve

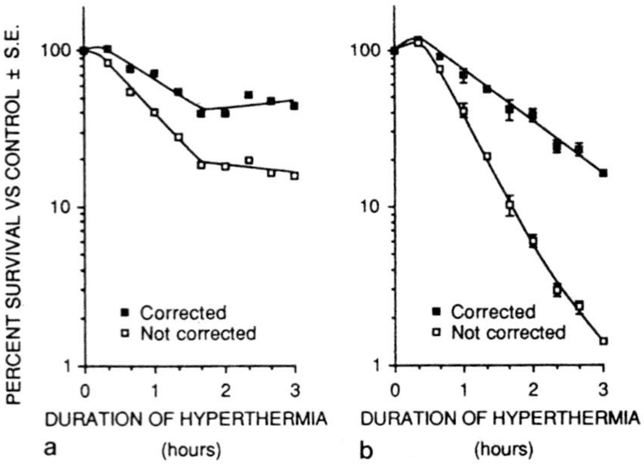

Fig. 10a, b. Thermal radiosensitization as a function of duration of pre-irradiation hyperthermia in JM (**a**) and MOLT3 (**b**) cells. Cells were heated at 41.5 °C for varying lengths of time immediately before receiving 4.0 Gy (JM) or 1.0 Gy (MOLT3) irradiation. Including time at 37.0 °C, all cell samples were incubated for 3 h. Survival was calculated as a percentage of the survival of irradiated, unheated controls with (■) and without (□) correcting for direct heat toxicity. *Bars*, SE (Cohen et al. 1988)

clinically meaningful radiosensitization. However, there is an obvious need for additional in vitro studies involving nonlymphoid neoplasms and other treatment sequences (i.e., hyperthermia after irradiation), and especially for in vivo studies designed to replicate potential clinical treatment scenarios (e.g., see Steeves et al. 1987).

The sequence of heating and irradiation could also have important clinical implications. It is often suggested that thermal radiosensitization is greatest when these agents are given simultaneously and that radiosensitization decreases sharply as the interval between heat and irradiation increases (Dewey 1984; Dewey et al. 1977a; Gillette and Ensley 1979; Li and Kal 1977; Robinson and Wizenberg 1974; Sapareto et al. 1978b, 1979). This generalization conjures up awkward images of attempting to simultaneously heat and irradiate a patient or having to rush patients between the hyperthermia facility and the radiotherapy center.

Fortunately, recent data suggest that an interval of perhaps even several hours can separate these two modalities and still produce supraadditive tumoricidal interactions. Indeed, such sequential combinations might actually provide a better therapeutic index than would simultaneous treatments.

Stating that simultaneous exposure will maximize radiosensitization greatly oversimplifies a complex subject. In reality, different types of malignant cells have different thermal sensitivities in vitro, they develop different degrees of thermal radiosensitization (Dewey et al. 1977a; Raaphorst et al. 1971), and they experience maximal radiosensitization with different heat-irradiation sequences and intervals. Cell killing may be maximal with heating before or during irradiation (Li and Kal 1977; Sapareto et al. 1978a), with heating during or after irradiation (Cohen et al. 1988; Li and Kal 1977) or when heating ends several hours before irradiation (Cohen et al. 1988). In some cell lines radiosensitization rapidly decreases if even short intervals (e.g., 5–10 min [Sapareto et al. 1978a]) at 37 °C are allowed between heat and irradiation (Dewey 1984; Raaphorst et al. 1983; Sapareto et al. 1978a). Sometimes little synergism is evident with intervals longer than 1–2 h (Sapareto et al. 1978a, 1979). However, in most cell lines thermal radiosensitization remains even if at least several hours elapse between heat and irradiation (e.g., Overgaard and Nielson 1983; even at 41.5 °C [Cohen et al. 1988]). In some cells, thermal radiosensitization occurs to an equal extent regardless of the sequence and interval used (Bromer et al. 1982; Raaphorst et al. 1983; Robinson et al. 1974; Steeves et al. 1987). For example, radiosensitivity is constant when MOLT 4 (a human T cell lymphoid malignancy) is treated in any sequence with 1.0 Gy and given 42.0 °C hyperthermia for 1 h (Raaphorst et al. 1983). The same occurs using other radiation doses (1.0–3.0 Gy) and at various higher temperatures up to 45.0 °C (for 5 min) (Raaphorst et al. 1983). Clearly, it is not possible to suggest an optimal general treatment sequence that would apply to all tumor types.

It is equally difficult to prescribe an ideal sequence and interval for a given *type* of tumor as even very similar cell lines can exhibit qualitatively different behaviors (Cohen et al. 1988). As an example, we might consider JM, MOLT 3, MOLT 4 – three human, T cell, acute lymphoblastic leukemia cell lines which have very similar nutritional requirements and proliferation rates in vitro (Cohen et al. 1988; Raaphorst et al. 1983). Synergism is maximal in JM cells when heat (41.5 °C for 1 h) is given 2–6 h before irradiation and is clearly less when heat and irradiation are given at the same time (Fig. 11) (Cohen et al. 1988). In MOLT 3, it is best to give heat (41.5 °C for 1 h) during or up to 4 h after irradiation (Fig. 12, Cohen et al. 1988). In MOLT 4, radiosensitization is not affected by heat-irradiation sequencing (42.0 °C) as we previously noted (Raaphorst et al. 1983). The profound distinctions between these three nearly identical cell lines serve as a reminder to be cautious when drawing general conclusions from observations made in just one cell line.

Regardless of how sequencing affects a particular cell line, increasing the treatment temperature or decreasing the pH lengthens the interval which can be allowed between heat and irradiation while still exhibiting supraadditive killing (Dewey et al. 1977a, Freeman et al. 1981; Gerweck et al. 1975; Holahan et al. 1984; Miyakoshi et al. 1982). For example, the data in Figs. 11 and 12 show that greater degrees of heat injury (in this instance due to higher temperatures) increase the amount of time required for thermal radiosensitization to return to normal in human lymphoblastic leukemia cell lines (Cohen et al. 1988). In the same way, for a given heat exposure, a longer interval is also required for synergism to resolve when cells are heated in S phase compared to other cells (Sapareto et al. 1978b). This is interesting as S phase is the most heat-sensitive cell cycle compartment (based on heating *at 45 °C* [Westra and Dewey 1971]).

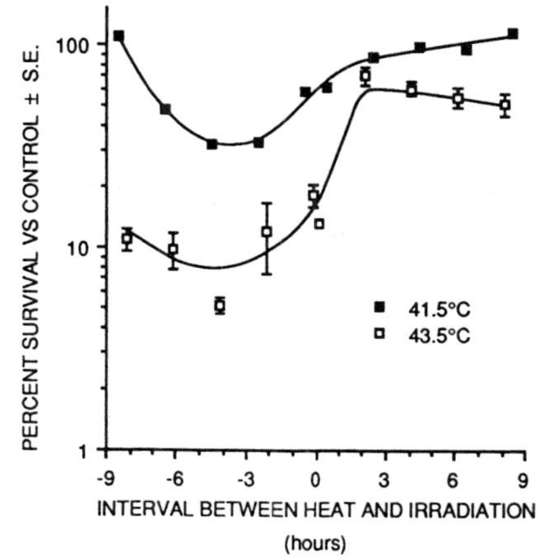

Fig. 11. Heat-irradiation sequence and survival of JM cells. Cells were heated for 1 h at 41.5 °C or for 20 min at 43.5 °C at varying times before (negative time values) and after (positive time values) irradiation to 4.0 Gy. *Points* indicate midpoints of heat exposures. Survival was corrected for direct heat killing and expressed as a percentage of the survival of unheated, irradiated controls. Less than 100% survival indicates thermal radiosensitization. *Bars*, SE

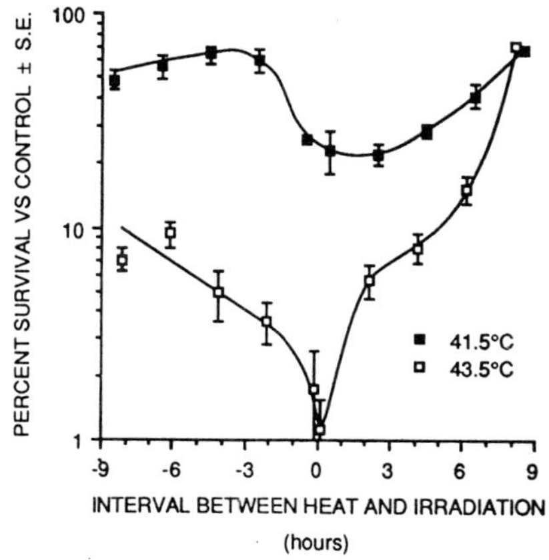

Fig. 12. Heat-irradiation sequence and survival of MOLT 3 cells. Procedures were as in Fig. 11 for JM cells except cells received 2.0 Gy irradiation. *Bars*, SE. (Cohen et al. 1988)

At least a group of studies suggests the possibility that treatment sequencing might also affect the duration of the radiosensitization effects (Overgaard 1980; Overgaard and Nielson 1983). In this study the radiosensitization effect lasted only a few hours when *normal* tissues were irradiated before heating (42.5 °C). In contrast, the same sequence produced a long period of radiosensitization in neoplastic cells (up to 24 h). As a result, the therapeutic index might be increased by intentionally allowing several hours between heat and irradiation – at least for this particular cell line (Overgaard and Nielson 1983).

The therapeutic index of combination therapy could also be improved by taking advantage of the positive correlation between thermal injury and the duration of the radiosensitization effect, a phenomenon which has been demonstrated repeatedly in a variety of cell lines (see above). Supraadditive killing should be greater and radiosensitization should persist longer in nutritionally deprived neoplastic cells than in surrounding normal tissues (see above). As a result, *with regard to the radiation-resistant nutritionally deprived tumor cells with which we are most concerned*, intentionally allowing an interval between heat and irradiation could improve radiation's therapeutic index.

Therapeutic gain factors have actually been calculated for various treatment sequences. In one study (Gillette and Ensley 1979) therapeutic gain factors of 1.2 – 1.3 were obtained for 30 min of heating (42.5 ° or 43 °C) for any heat-irradiation sequence, when 15 min of heating was given 2 h before or during irradiation or when irradiation preceded 1 h of hyperthermia. Interestingly, for 15 and 60 min of heating, the other treatment sequences that were tested gave no apparent therapeutic gain (Gillette and Ensley 1979). Although these temperatures might not be relevant to the setting of systemic hyperthermia, it is an interesting observation that the therapeutic gain varied in a complex manner with changes in heating temperature, heating duration and sequence. Parenthetically, it should also be noted that 42.5 °C at least approaches the WBH range and the above results are comparable to therapeutic gain factors of 1.21 – 1.75 when 41 °C and 42 °C local hyperthermia (for 1 h) and irradiation were given simultaneously (Robinson et al. 1974).

Thermal tolerance, a temporary resistance to heat killing that is induced by a prior heat exposure, *might* also influence the development of thermal radiosensitization (Nielsen et al. 1983). In particular, it has been suggested that radiosensitivity decreases when thermal tolerance develops after heating at ≥42.5 °C (Holahan et al. 1984; Overgaard 1984; Raaphorst and Azzam 1983; van Rijn et al. 1984). It happens, however, that the relationship between thermal tolerance and radiosensitivity has not yet been clearly established even for temperatures above 42.5 °C – the temperature range in the majority of thermal tolerance studies. Sometimes thermal tolerance has no discermable effect on the magnitude of thermal radiosensitization (Bromer et al. 1982; Cohen et al. 1988; Mivechi and Li 1987; Nielson 1983; Steeves et al. 1987).

The impact of thermal tolerance *at this higher temperature range* is further obscured by evidence that thermal tolerance also develops in normal tissues (Urano 1986) and that thermal tolerance occurs and resolves at different rates in different tissues and cell lines (Holahan et al. 1984; Jorritsma et al. 1985; Overgaard 1984; Raaphorst and Azzam 1983; van Rijn et al. 1984). In addition, significantly less thermal tolerance develops at lower pH, an interesting effect which suggests the possibility that tumor might be disproportionately injured by fractionated radiotherapy-hyperthermia schedules which induce thermal tolerance in normal tissues (Goldin and Leeper 1981; Holahan et al. 1984; Nielson and Overgaard 1979). It is also possible that thermal tolerance is a small consideration (in regard to thermal radiosensitization) compared to other factors such as pH or net thermal injury (Holahan et al. 1984). Because of these many considerations it is very difficult to confidently estimate the *cumulative* impact of thermal tolerance (at >42.5 °C) on the therapeutic index of radiotherapy. Conceivably, different experimental temperatures might explain the divergent findings of some thermal tolerance studies (Raaphorst and Azzam 1983). More specifically, there is at least some evidence that thermal tolerance might have little or no impact on thermal radiosensitization in the WBH temperature range. For example, the C3H mammary carcinoma cell line develops marked, prolonged thermal tolerance after treatments at temperatures above 42.5 °C. However, 42.5 °C has a relatively small and brief thermal tolerance effect (Overgaard 1984) and it is not clear whether clinically relevant thermal tolerance would be seen at 41.8 °C.

In another study radiant heat WBH (41.5 ° ±0.5 °C for 1 h for 4 consecutive days) with TBI (1 Gy per day for 4 days) significantly increased survival of leukemia-bearing AKR mice without any apparent interference by thermal tolerance ($p = 0.0001$, compared to controls treated with single modality WBH or irradiation) (Steeves et al. 1987). This was the case even when the target temperature was intentionally reached slowly to increase the probability that thermal tolerance might become manifest (Steeves et al. 1987). Studies like these using *systemic hyperthermia temperatures* suggest that thermal tolerance either does not develop

4 WBH and Chemotherapy

4.1 Introduction

Temperatures compatible with WBH can profoundly enhance the cytotoxic actions of many commonly used chemotherapeutic drugs. In addition, some compounds which are not cytotoxic at normal body temperature have supraadditive cytotoxic interactions with hyperthermia. These agents have been variously termed "labilizers" or "thermal sensitizers" (see Robins et al. 1983d, 1984a).

Because of technological and conceptual factors, the investigation of these various agents has proceeded in two phases. The first phase concentrated almost exclusively on demonstrating which drugs exhibit supraadditive tumoricidal interactions with hyperthermia in vitro and then in vivo. Presently, representative compounds from most clinically important drug classes have been studied. These findings are summarized in this chapter in a series of tables. Some of the better known labilizing drugs are also considered. The second phase has involved clarifying (a) whether hyperthermia produces a therapeutic gain for various drugs (i.e., increases the killing of cancer cells relative to the killing of normal cells), and (b) which variables affect the magnitude of the therapeutic index. Although some work has been done in this area, in many ways this second phase is still in its infancy as is discussed later in the chapter.

Studies of thermal chemosensitization are complicated by pharmacologic concerns which are less prominent or sometimes even nonexistent problems in thermal radiosensitization. Heat alters multiple physiologic and biochemical processes which have implications for drug pharmacokinetics, cellular drug permeability or uptake, drug activation, metabolism and excretion. A consideration of the experience with cyclophosphamide will illustrate some of the types of issues which arise.

Studies involving cyclophosphamide have been complicated by the parent compound's need for hepatic activation. Consequently, there has been a heavy dependence on in vivo experimental systems (Dahl and Mella 1983; Hazan et al. 1981; Hiramoto et al. 1984; Honess and Bleehan 1982; Longo et al. 1983; Murray et al. 1984; Urano and Kim 1983; West et al. 1980), or the use of organ level studies involving extracorporeal liver sections or isolated liver perfusion (Clawson et al. 1981; Collins and Skibba 1983). Most in vivo tumor models rely on end points such as tumor volume doubling times (Haas et al. 1984; Longo et al. 1983; Senapati et al. 1982), tumor growth delay (Dahl and Mella 1983; Hazan et al. 1984; Urano and Kim 1983), tumor regression (Dahl and Mella 1983; Malangoni et al. 1978; West et al. 1980), animal survival (Haas et al. 1984; Lorenz et al. 1983; Malangoni et al. 1978; Rose et al. 1979; Yerushalmi and Hazan 1979), or cure rate (Hazan et al. 1981; Yerushalmi and Hazan 1979). Such end points are not optimally sensitive or specific with regard to clearly distinguishing between supraadditive and merely additive cytotoxic interactions. In vivo quantification of individual cellular survival, such as using spleen colony or lung colony formation, would be greatly preferable. For the example of cyclophosphamide, actual cellular survival of normal and neoplastic cells appears to have been addressed only by Honess and Bleehan (Honess and Bleehan 1982). Almost all in vivo studies have also shown a strong preference for local or regional hyperthermia with rather few investigators using WBH (e.g., Honess and Bleehan 1982, 1985a; Honess et al. 1985; Rose et al. 1979; Rotstein et al. 1983; Tapozoglou et al. 1988; Thuning et al. 1980). The physiologic effects of local-regional methods can be quite different from those of WBH as is discussed in Chap. 5 (as is also discussed in Chap 5 – toxicities and physiologic effects vary even between different WBH technologies). To give just one hypothetical example, different methods could have different effects on hepatic metabolic function (Clawson et al. 1981; Collins and Skibba 1983), and presumably also on hepatic vascular perfusion as well as on renal perfusion and excretion. In this way, the type of hyperthermia system being used and the hepatic temperature distribution could significantly influence the activation and excretion of many drugs. The data in Fig. 1 (Mella 1985) exemplify these types of concerns. Cisplatin plus local hyperthermia

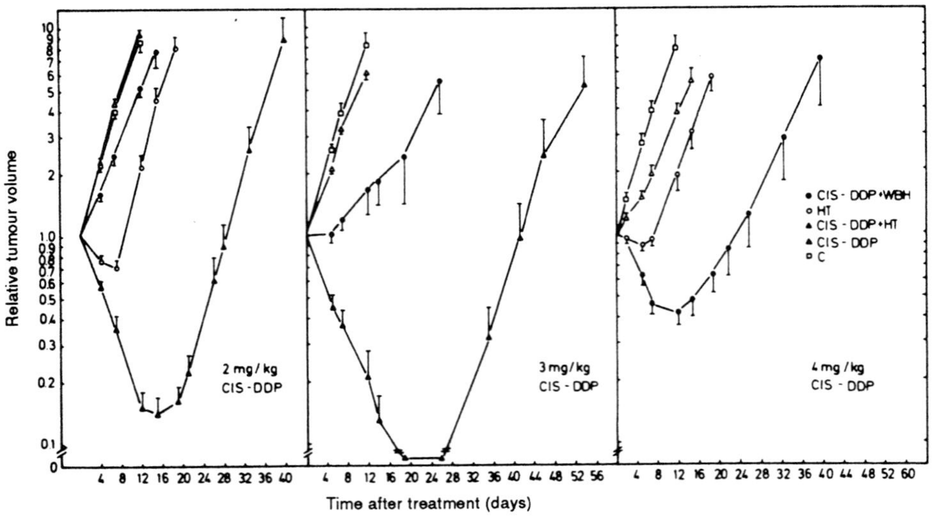

Fig. 1. Growth curves of groups of similarly treated BR_4A tumors in three separate experiments. A growth curve is not drawn for cisplatin (CIS-DDP), 4 mg/kg and hyperthermia of the tumor-bearing leg (HT), as there were permanent tumor controls. Each *point* is the mean of at least five tumors. *WBH*, whole body hyperthermia by immersing the nontumor-bearing leg in the waterbath. *Vertical bars*, ±SEM (Mella 1985)

(water bath immersion of the tumor-bearing leg) gives a substantially different result than does cisplatin plus WBH (induced by immersion of the nontumor-bearing leg).

Experiments with nitrosoureas exemplify several other considerations. With these drugs, temperature elevation significantly accelerates drug hydrolysis and also drug inactivation due to serum protein binding (e.g., Hahn 1978). Thus, heat increases cytotoxicity *per unit of available active drug* while simultaneously acting to decrease the active drug concentration. Perhaps for these reasons, some early studies reported little or no thermal chemosensitization for these agents (Hahn 1974). However, thermal enhancement was apparent for nitrosoureas when subsequent experiments were carefully corrected to address actual *active* drug concentrations as a function of time (Hahn 1978).

Nonchemotherapeutic drugs given to animals during hyperthermia can introduce other unexpected effects. For example, one study combined melphalan and 41.44 °–42 °C hyperthermia (water bath immersion) in the treatment of B16 melanoma and Lewis lung carcinoma tumors (Joiner et al. 1982). Thermal enhancement ratios of 1.55 and 2.43 were observed for the two tumor types respectively. However, dose modifying factors of 1.78 and 2.69 were also measured in sham-treated animals which were anesthetized but not heated (Joiner et al. 1982). An example of such a re-

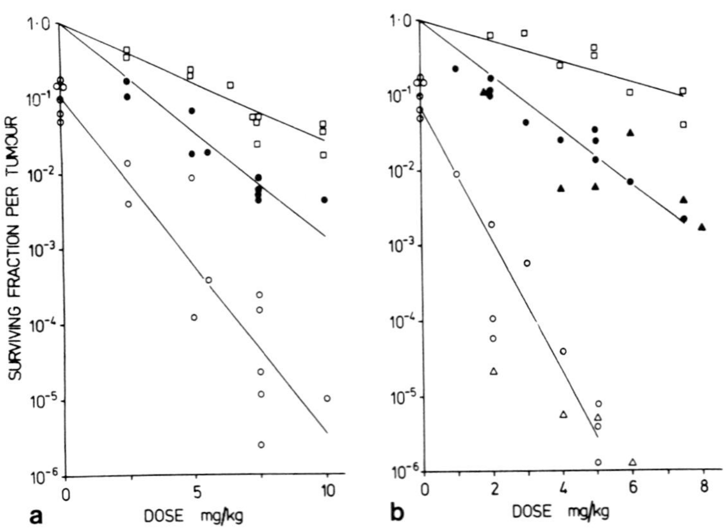

Fig. 2 a, b. Cell survival in Lewis lung carcinoma 24 h after treatment with **a** CCNU or **b** melphalan. Unheated tumors in conscious mice (□); unheated tumors in mice anesthetized by Saffan (●) or Sagatal (▲); heated tumors (43 °C for 1 h) in mice anesthetized by Saffan (○) or Sagatal (△). (Joiner et al. 1982)

sult is shown in Fig. 2 for lomustine (CCNU) and melphalan (Joiner et al. 1982).

In similar studies, local anesthetics including lidocaine, procaine, butacaine, tetracaine, and dibucaine enhanced the cytotoxicity of peplomycin, a bleomycin derivative, in the FM3A murine mammary adenocarcinoma and in HeLa cells in vitro (Mizuno and Ishida 1982). Ethanol enhanced leomycin killing (Mizuno 1981; Mizuno and Ishida 1981) as did lidocaine (Lazo et al. 1985). Similarly, lidocaine enhanced doxorubicin cytotoxicity (Chlebowski et al. 1982). Collectively, these observations are consistent with the view that local anesthetics and ethanol might enhance bleomycin or doxorubicin killing by affecting the structure or permeability of cellular membranes (Mizuno and Ishida 1982; Chlebowski et al. 1982). Interestingly, however, the same anesthetic agents did not similarly enhance killing by mitomycin C or cisplatin (Mizuno and Ishida 1982), and ethanol did not enhance doxorubicin or cisplatin killing (Mizuno and Ishida 1981, 1982). This suggests that chemotherapeutic drugs must be considered on an individual basis. In a more general sense, such studies show that it is clearly necessary to control for possible effects of "adjunctive" drugs when designing in vivo hyperthermia experiments. Concern about these sorts of confounding interactions was one of the motives behind the recent development of WBH techniques for unrestrained, unanesthetized animals (Robins et al. 1984c).

As a final precautionary note, it should also be remembered that the results of thermal chemosensitization studies can strongly vary depending on the cell line being used. In one of the best examples, sensitization to melphalan in seven melanoma cell lines varied widely all the way from no thermal sensitization to marked enhancement (Goss and Parsons 1977). We have also observed significant variability in the magnitude of thermal sensitization (carboplatin) in two extremely similar human T cell acute lymphoblastic leukemia cell lines (Cohen and Robins 1987; Cohen et al. 1989b). As is shown in Fig. 3 (Wallner et al. 1987) the dose enhancement ratio at a given temperature can differ even between various sublines of a single cell line, e.g., the HA-1 parent line and its mitomycin C resistant clones HA-M3 and HA-M4 (see also Rofstad and Brustad 1985). Altogether, it is not clear how often thermal chemosensitization varies between different cell lines. However, it is quite clear that experiments involving even very similar cell lines can give quite different results under identical conditions. As a result, it is necessary to be skeptical of general-

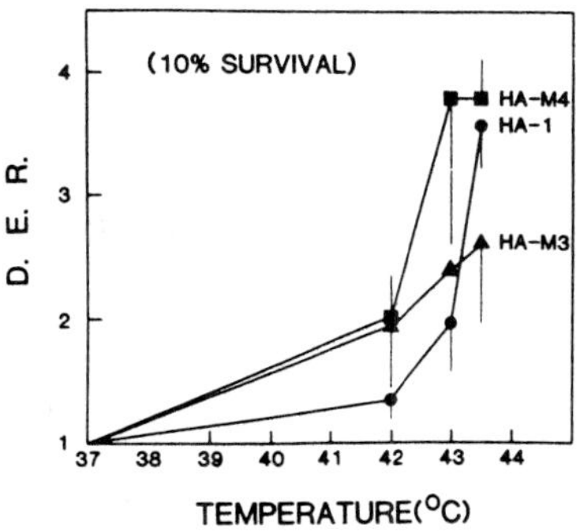

Fig. 3. Dose enhancement ratios (D.E.R.) at 42°, 43°, and 43.5°C. Calculations were made after correction for heat killing. *Bars*, SE. (Wallner et al. 1987)

Table 1. Extensively studied, clinically applicable chemotherapeutic drugs which have supraadditive tumoricidal interactions with hyperthermia[a]

Drug	In vitro studies	In vivo studies
Alkylating agents		
Cyclophosphamide		+ (Collins and Skibba 1983; Dahl and Mella 1983; Haas et al. 1984; Hazan et al. 1981, 1984; Hiramoto et al. 1984; **Honess and Bleehan 1982**; Longo et al. 1983; Loven et al. 1986; Malangoni et al. 1978; Murray et al. 1984; Senapati et al. 1982; Urano and Kim 1983; West et al. 1980; Yerushalmi and Hazan 1979) − (Lorenz et al. 1983; Rose et al. 1979)
Mechlorethamine		+ (Collins and Skibba 1979; Kamura et al. 1979; Kremkau et al. 1976; Shingleton et al. 1962)
Melphalan	+ (Goss and Parsons 1977; Neumann et al. 1985)	+ (**Honess and Bleehan 1985a, b**; Joiner et al. 1982; Senapati et al. 1982)

Table 1 (continued)

Drug	In vitro studies	In vivo studies
Nitrosoureas (principally BCNU and CCNU)	+ (Barranco et al. 1975; Hahn 1978, 1979, 1983; Hahn and Shiu 1983; Herman et al. 1982a)	+ (Dahl and Mella 1982; **Honess and Bleehan 1982**; Joiner et al. 1982; Li and Hahn 1984; Marmor 1979; O'Donnell et al. 1979; Thuning et al. 1980; Twentyman et al. 1978) – **(Rose et al. 1979)**
Thiotepa	+ (Johnson and Pavlec 1973)	+ (Mahaley and Woodhall 1961; Longo et al. 1983)
Antitumor antibiotics or their analogues		
Actinomycin D	+ (Donaldson et al. 1978; Mizuno et al. 1980; Neumann et al. 1985)	+ (**Rose et al. 1979**; Yerushalmi 1978)
Bleomycin	+ (Braun and Hahn 1975; Fujiwara et al. 1984; Hahn 1974; Hahn et al. 1975; Hahn and Shiu 1983; Kubota et al. 1979; Ishida and Mizuno 1982; Lin et al. 1983a, b; Mizuno and Ishida 1981; Mizuno et al. 1980; Morgan et al. 1979; Morgan and Bleehan 1981a, b; Nakajima and Hisazumi 1983; Neumann et al. 1985; Roizin-Towle and Hall 1982)	+ (Dahl and Mella 1982; Hahn et al. 1975; Hassanzadeh and Chapman 1983; Li and Hahn 1984; Magan et al. 1979; Marmor 1979; Szcepanski and Trott 1981; Urano et al. 1988)
Doxorubicin	+ (Adwankar and Chitnis 1984; Chlebowski et al. 1982; Dahl and Mella 1982; Hahn et al. 1975; Hahn and Strande 1976; Hahn 1979; Herman 1983b; Li and Hahn 1978; Mizuno et al. 1980; Mizuno and Ishida 1982; Morgan et al. 1979; Morgan and Bleehan 1981a; Neumann et al. 1985; Roizin-Towle and Hall 1982) – (Li 1984; Li and Hahn 1984)	+ (Dahl 1983; Haas et al. 1984; Kamura et al. 1979; Magin et al. 1980; Overgaard 1976) – (Marmor 1979; **Rotstein et al. 1983**)
Mitomycin C	+ (Barlogie et al. 1980; Mizuno et al. 1980; Mizuno and Ishida 1982; Teicher et al. 1981b)	+ (Haas et al. 1984; Kamura et al. 1979; Koga et al. 1984)
Mitoxantrone	+ (Herman 1983a; Ohnoshi et al. 1985; Yang and Rafla 1985)	
Platinum compounds		
Carboplatin	+ (Cohen and Robins 1987; Cohen et al. 1989a, b, 1990; Cohen and Robins 1990b)	+ **(Tapazoglou et al. 1988; Page et al. 1989)**
Cisplatin	+ (Barlogie et al. 1980; Cohen et al. 1989a; Fisher and Hahn 1982; Hahn 1979; Herman et al. 1982a; Klein et al. 1977; Meyn et al. 1980; Neumann et al. 1985; Roizin-Towle and Hall 1982)	+ (Alberts et al. 1980; Douple et al. 1982; Haas et al. 1984; Hazan et al. 1984; **Mella 1985**; Wile et al. 1983a)

+, presence; or –, absence of supraadditive tumoricidal interactions between hyperthermia and drug.
[a] Studies which involve WBH in at least some measure are highlighted in bold type.

izations based on studies involving only a few cell lines.

This last observation partly explains our decision to list in Table 1 those drugs for which *multiple*, largely consistent studies exist. We have also tried to focus on drugs which are in active clinical use and have attempted to list most of the available major articles. Several negative studies are included in Table 1 primarily to emphasize that there is not complete concordance between all experimental systems. As we have commented, some variability in results might simply reflect the use of different cell lines or heating methods, etc. In addition, some experiments were conducted in such a manner that thermal enhancement might not have been expected. For example, in some cases an extremely long interval was allowed between heating and drug administration (e.g., 1 and 8 days [Lorenz et al. 1983]). In other instances, heating might not have been long enough (e.g., only 20 min [Rose et al. 1979]) or especially low temperatures were employed (e.g., 38.8°–38.9 °C for 45 min [Rose et al. 1979]), as is suggested by the fact that other investiga-

tors observed enhancement for the same cell line using higher temperatures of 42.6° and 42 °C (Hazan et al. 1981; Yerushalmi and Hazan 1979).
Table 2 lists drugs for which thermal chemosensitization probably occurs but for which relatively few studies are available.

Table 2. Less extensively studied, clinically applicable chemotherapeutic drugs[a]

Drug	In vitro studies	In vivo studies
Dacarbazine	+ (Mann et al. 1983)	– (Orth et al. 1977)
Daunorubicin	– (Mizuno et al. 1980)	
5-Fluorouracil	+ (Joshi and Barendsen 1984; Lange et al. 1984; Mini et al. 1986) – (Joshi and Barendsen 1984; Mizuno et al. 1980)	– (Adwankar and Chitnis 1984; Kamura et al. 1979)
Ifosfamide	+ (Fujiwara et al. 1984)	
Methotrexate	– (Herman et al. 1981) – (Hahn and Shiu 1983)	– (Muckle and Dickson 1973)
Procarbazine		+ (Senapati et al. 1982)
Tetraplatin	+ (Cohen and Robins 1990)	

+, presence; or –, absence of supraadditive tumoricidal interactions between hyperthermia and drug.
[a] Use of bold type as described for Table 1.

Table 3. Chemotherapeutic drugs which do not appear to have supraadditive tumoricidal interactions with hyperthermia

Drug	In vitro studies	In vivo studies
Etoposide	– (Cohen et al. 1989a)	
m-AMSA	– (Herman 1983a)	
Cytosine arabinoside	– (Adwankar and Chitnis 1984; Mizuno et al. 1980)	
Vincristine	+ (Adwankar and Chitnis 1984) – (Mizuno et al. 1980)	
Vindesine	– (Herman 1983a)	
Vinblastine	– (Joshi and Barendsen 1984; Neumann et al. 1985)	

+, presence; or –, absence of supraadditive tumoricidal interactions between hyperthermia and drug.

Table 3 lists those agents for which thermal sensitization probably does not occur or for which hyperthermia may actually even decrease antineoplastic efficacy.

4.2 Potential Mechanisms of Thermal Chemosensitization

Cytotoxic drugs for which thermal sensitization occurs appear to kill cells by a variety of mechanisms which generally can be described as (a) chemically interacting with and damaging DNA, or (b) disrupting DNA precursor synthesis. Despite the ability to make such generalizations, primary molecular events and their sequelae differ from drug to drug. Also, many compounds simultaneously induce several potentially harmful types of lesions as is discussed in most general oncology texts. As an example, alkylation of basis by alkylating agents can result in DNA strand breakage, misreading errors, and eventually inhibition of DNA, RNA, and protein synthesis (Ludlum 1977). "Bifunctional" alkylating agents can also cause interstrand and intrastrand crosslinking (Kohn 1977).
Conceivably, therefore, hyperthermia might affect the primary drug-DNA reaction and/or any of the secondary consequences of this primary interaction. Thus, despite the obvious mechanistic similarities between different drugs, we view each compound as a world "world unto itself" offering multiple, sometimes unique opportunities for thermal sensitization. Unfortunately, for no drug has there ever been a truly exhaustive investigation of all the reasonably plausible thermal chemosensitization mechanisms, i.e., a careful evaluation of all reasonable possibilities. Instead, numerous independent studies offer isolated glimpses into possible mechanisms. Because of the uncoordinated, scattered nature of the available studies, it is best to simply compile the available mechanistic information. If it achieves nothing else, this approach supports the view that (a) there are common motifs which apply to many drugs, and (b) thermal sensitization may involve multiple mechanisms for a given drug.
Several of the most plausible proposed mechanisms involve simple physicochemical consequences of heat such as accelerated drug activation and drug-DNA interactions. Thermal enhancement of thiotepa killing, for instance, may relate to increased formation of ethylenimine radicals or accelerated alkylation (Johnson and Pavelec 1973). As is shown in Fig. 4 (Teicher et al. 1981a), activation of mitomycin C to an alkylating species is increased at elevated temperatures. For

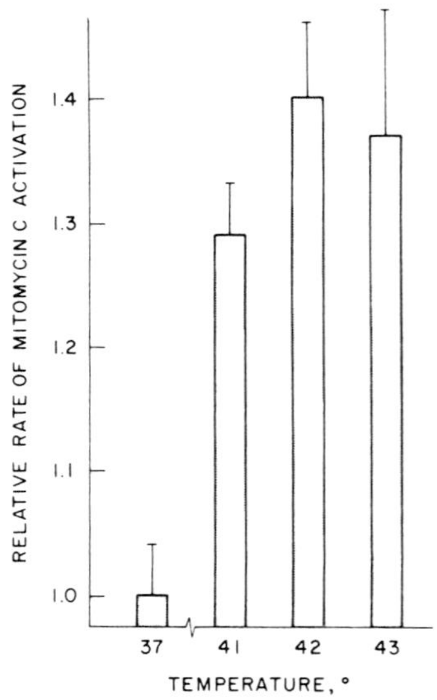

Fig. 4. Relative rate of activation of mitomycin C to an alkylating species by EMT6 cell-free preparations under anaerobic conditions at different temperatures. The alkylating species generated from mitomycin C was trapped and quantitated using 4-(*p*-nitrobenzyl)pyridine (Teicher et al. 1981 b)

other drugs, such as mechlorethamine, both degradation and reactivity may be increased by simultaneous heating (Collins and Skibba 1979). Heat appears to accelerate nitrosourea hydrolysis and possibly alkylation (De Silva et al. 1985; Hahn 1978). Similar results have been observed regarding cisplatin activation (Riviere et al. 1986).

Another physical effect of heat might be changes in membrane permeability and accelerated cellular drug uptake (Magin and Niesman 1984). For example, hyperthermia increases cellular doxorubicin entry in vitro (Hahn and Strande 1976; Mizuno and Ishida 1982) as is shown in Fig. 5 (Bates and MacKillop 1989). Hyperthermia may also modestly increase cellular methotrexate uptake (e.g., 30%) especially into cells which exhibit little or no active methotrexate uptake (Herman et al. 1981). In vivo, muscle tissue uptake of radiolabelled mechlorethamine was greater at 41 °–43 °C than at 30 °–32 °C in dogs (Shingleton et al. 1962). In rabbits, the drug was preferentially taken up into VX2 carcinoma tissue compared to drug uptake into adjacent normal tissue (Shingleton et al. 1962). Similarly, in another hyperthermia study, cisplatin cytotoxicity and also cellular drug levels were greater for P388 leukemia than for normal marrow cells (Alberts et al. 1980). (Other studies have not observed the same potentially advantageous differential uptake with cisplatin [Honess 1983; Neumann et al. 1985] although both "negative" studies may have employed inadequate temperatures, i.e., 41 °C [Honess 1983] or 40.5 °C [Neumann et al. 1985]). In vivo observations of increased tissue drug levels may be partly related to pharmacokinetic changes. For instance, in one investigations hyperthermia increased not only peak tumor melphalan levels but also peak serum levels (Honess et al. 1985).

It should be pointed out that increases in cellular drug levels sometimes appear inadequate to completely account for the observed thermal enhancement. For example, hyperthermia increased membrane permeability to melphalan in Chinese hamster ovary cells in vitro, resulting in greater drug uptake *and* egress (Bates and MacKillop 1989). Overall, there was a net 20% increase in steady state cellular drug levels. This increase by itself seems incongruous with the fourfold increase in cytotoxicity which was observed. For other drugs such as bleomycin, there is reasonable evidence that thermal enhancement can occur without accompanying increases in cellular drug uptake (Braun and Hahn 1975; Lin et al. 1983 a).

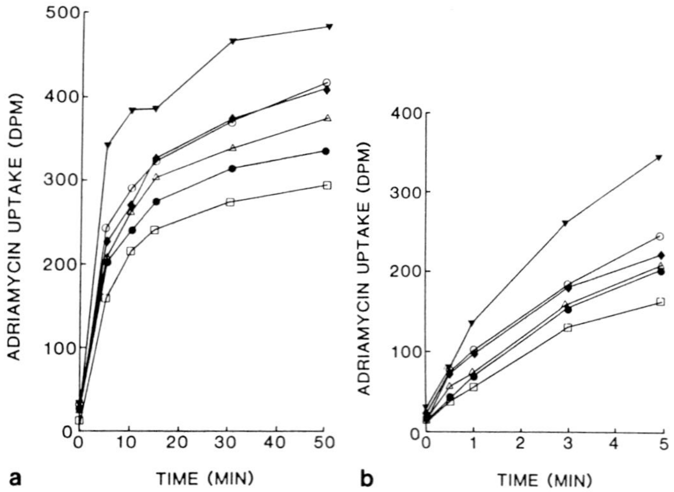

Fig. 5 a, b. Time courses for temperature dependence of Adriamycin uptake. Reaction mixtures containing 10^6 CHO cells and Adriamycin (1 μg/ml) were heated for times up to either **a** 50 min or **b** 5 min in 0.2 ml phosphate-buffered saline (PBS), 1% bovine serum albumin (BSA), 10 m*M* glucose with pH 7.4 at 31 °C (□), 37 °C (●), 40 °C (△), 43 °C (♦), 45 °C (○), and 50 °C (▼). Means are given for 9–18 estimations from 3–5 separate experiments. (Bares and MacKillop 1987)

A comparable study illustrates the problems inherent in assuming a simple relationship between one measure of drug activity/uptake and drug cytotoxicity. In this instance, heating increased net cisplatin-DNA adduct formation (Meyn et al. 1980). Cytotoxicity increased tenfold while DNA adducts increased 6.5-fold (Meyn et al. 1980). This observation has been interpreted as evidence that thermal enhancement is not fully explained by increased DNA adduct formation. However, it may simply be that cytotoxicity correlates with adduct formation in a nonlinear manner. Thus, for this experimental system, increased adduct formation might fully account for thermal enhancement of cisplatin toxicity.

In at least some experimental systems, thermal enhancement occurs even if drugs are given after heating ends (e.g., bleomycin [Braun and Hahn 1975], carboplatin [Cohen and Robins 1987], cisplatin [Corry et al. 1984; Wallner and Li 1987], or thiotepa [Longo et al. 1983]). Indeed, in some cases thermal enhancement is essentially equivalent when heating immediately precedes drug exposure and when the two agents are given simultaneously (Cohen 1987; Corry et al. 1984; Wallner and Li 1987) and enhancement can be observed when heating ends as many as 5 h before drug exposure (Cohen and Robins 1987). It is possible that these observations result from hyperthermia-induced changes in membrane permeability which simply persist after heating ends. However, these sequencing studies provide evidence that heat has effects besides just its direct physical acceleration of drug activation and drug-DNA reaction rates. The ability of *43 °C* hyperthermia to decrease bleomycin degrading enzyme activity may be one example of such a possible alternative mechanism (Lin et al. 1983 a, b). Similarly, it has been suggested that hyperthermia may enhance methotrexate toxicity (to the extent that enhancement of methotrexate killing really occurs) by reducing intracellular dihydrofolate reductase activity (Herman et al. 1981).

There have been repeated suggestions that heat may inhibit DNA repair (e.g., Hahn et al. 1975; Kubota et al. 1979; Meyn et al. 1980). Possibly this may be viewed as an extension of the idea of heat inactivating key cellular enzymes of otherwise reducing their activity. There is also evidence that hyperthermia decreases the availability of key substrates for some enzymes involved in DNA repair. For example, Robins et al. have observed that hyperthermia significantly reduces NAD^+ pools in human peripheral blood lymphocytes. This applies to lymphocytes heated in vitro as well as to lymphocytes from patients undergoing WBH. NAD^+ ist the key, rate-limiting substrate for poly(ADP ribose) polymerase, an important enzyme involved in recovery from DNA injury. WBH also decreases cellular ATP which is used in regenerating NAD^+ (Robins et al. 1991 b).

Despite widespread enthusiasm for theories involving DNA repair, there is limited evidence that temperatures compatible with WBH actually have such effects (as with thermal radiosensitization discussed in Chap. 3). Specifically, there is only one suggestion that this might be the case, i.e., 41.5 °C hyperthermia decreased DNA repair for methyl methanesulfonate and 42 °C hyperthermia increased the formation of single-stranded DNA breaks in concert with increasing drug cytotoxicity (Bronk et al. 1973).

A final possibility is that cytokinetic effects of hyperthermia or drugs may help to explain some observations of thermal sensitization such as that seen between 5-FU and hyperthermia in one study (Mini et al. 1986). This possibility, which needs to be confirmed, is only applicable to 5-FU at this time.

The preceding discussion summarizes the types of processes which could be involved in thermal chemosensitization. These disparate observations are compatible with several reasonable scenarios. First, in studying a single cell line it is quite possible that one sensitization mechanism might predominate to the extent that it can account for nearly all of the observed enhancement effect (e.g., Meyn et al. 1980). In other cells it is quite possible that multiple processes might make detectable contributions. Analogous suggestions appear to be very reasonable with regard to an individual drug, i.e., one process may predominate or there may be several important phenomena.

4.3 Factors Which May Modify Thermal Chemosensitization

4.3.1 Heat-drug Sequence

The effect of heat-drug sequencing has been studied at least for actinomycin D (Donaldson et al. 1978), bleomycin (Braun and Hahn 1975; Lin et al. 1983 a, b; Mizuno and Ishida 1981; Nakajima and Hisazumi 1983; Szczepanski and Trott 1981), carboplatin (Cohen and Robins 1987), cisplatin (Baba et al. 1989; Corry et al. 1984; Fisher and Hahn 1982; Wallner et al. 1986; Wallner and Li 1987), cyclophosphamide (Dahl and Mella 1983; Dahl and Mella 1984; Urano and Kim 1983), doxorubicin (Hahn and Strande 1976), 5-FU (Mini et al. 1986), melphalan (Joiner et al. 1982), methotrexate (Herman et al. 1981), mitomycin C (Wallner et al. 1987), the nitrosoureas (Hahn 1979; Marmor 1979; O'Donnell et al. 1979), and

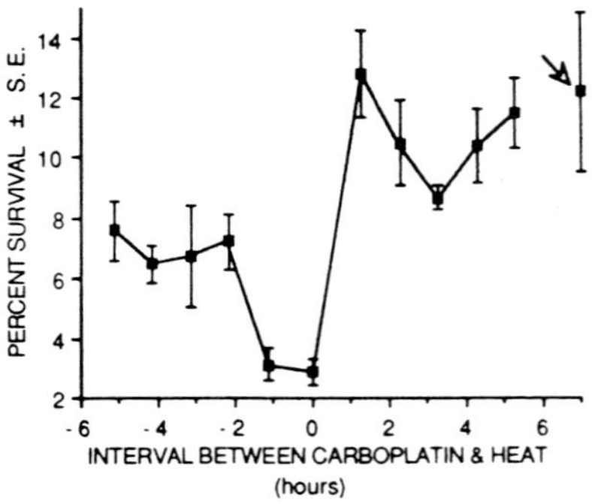

Fig. 6. Effect of treatment sequence on killing by heat and carboplatin. Cells were heated for 60 min at 41.8 °C at varying times before (negative time values), during (time 0), and after (positive time values) a 60-min carboplatin treatment at 60 µg/ml. Survival was calculated as a percentage of the survival of untreated controls and was corrected for direct heat killing. *Points*, midpoints of heat exposures; *arrow*, survival after carboplatin treatment alone at 37 °C (Cohen and Robins 1987)

thiotepa (Longo et al. 1983). Most of these studies have found that maximal thermal sensitization occurs when hyperthermia is applied during or shortly before drug exposure. An example of this effect is shown in Fig. 6 (Cohen and Robins 1987) for JM human leukemia cells treated with carboplatin. Alternatively, for HA-1 Chinese hamster fibroblast cells in vitro, heat was best given during or after mitomycin C as is shown in Fig. 7 (Wallner et al. 1987).

In most cell lines, as was mentioned previously, enhancement is apparent even with up to several hours separating the two modalities (e.g., Figs. 6 and 7). Similarly, there is evidence that BCNU cytotoxicity at 37 °C may be enhanced for as long as 24 h after a single 43 °C heat exposure (Hahn 1983; Morgan et al. 1979).

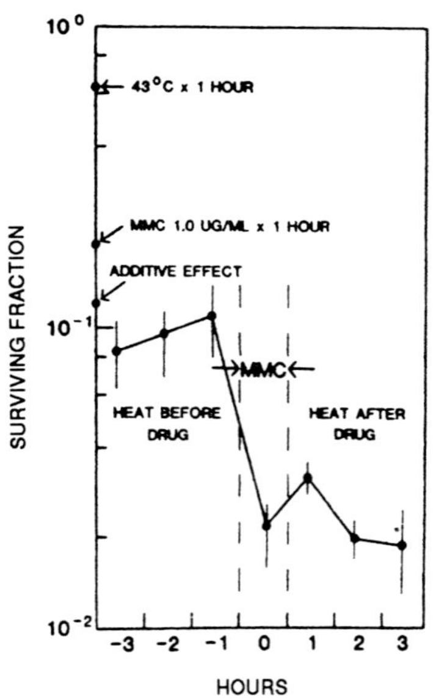

Fig. 7. Effect of sequencing on mitomycin C (*MMC*)-heat interaction in HA-1 cells. When heating was done after MMC exposure, cells were rinsed with phosphate-buffered saline and maintained at 37 °C in full medium until heating. Additive effect is derived by multiplying survival following heat alone (43 °C for 1 h) by survival following exposure to MMC alone (1.0 µg/ml) as described by Valeriote and Lin (12). *Bars*, SE; *U*, µ (Wallner et al. 1987)

4.3.2 Temperature

If hyperthermia enhances the cytotoxicity of a drug, the degree of enhancement generally increases with rising temperature (Cohen and Robins 1987; Engelhardt 1987; Hahn 1979; Herman et al. 1984a). In this regard, it has been suggested that many drugs can be grouped into (a) compounds for which thermal enhancement abruptly increases above a certain threshold temperature (doxorubicin, bleomycin), and (b) compounds for which there is no apparent threshold temperature, i.e., thermal sensitization gradually increases with rising temperatures (cisplatin, bifunctional alkylating agents, nitrosoureas) (Hahn 1982). This idea is quite intriguing as is the related notion that drugs in a given group might exhibit common mechanisms of thermal sensitization. Nevertheless, a note of caution is needed; in at least one instance this classification schema does not even allow generalization from one drug to other closely related compounds. For example, cisplatin is considered a prototypical drug for not exhibiting a sensitization threshold temperature (Hahn 1982). Yet, an abrupt threshold is readily apparent for carboplatin and tetraplatin

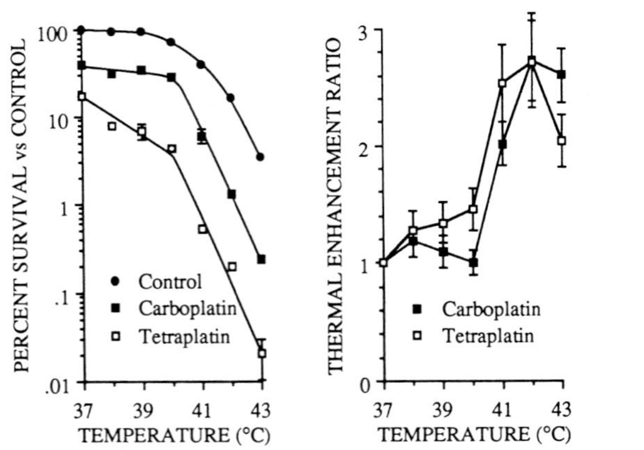

Fig. 8. Survival and thermal enhancement ratios for exponentially growing JM cells exposed to carboplatin (0 or 45 µg/ml) for 1 h at 37 °–43 °C in increments of 1 °C. Standard errors are encompassed in the symbols except when indicated by brackets (Cohen and Robins 1990b)

as is shown in Fig. 8 (Cohen and Robins 1990a, b) even though carboplatin and cisplatin have an identical active form (Cohen and Robins 1990). At the very least, this observation raises doubts about the idea that drugs in a given "threshold class" might exhibit similar thermal sensitization mechanisms.

This inconsistency brings to mind certain new hypotheses regarding sensitization threshold temperatures. Specifically, whether a given drug shows a threshold temperature might sometimes reflect the cell line chosen for the sensitization assay, e.g., for some cell lines, threshold effects might occur regardless of the "heat-sensitive" drug being tested whereas other cell lines might not exhibit threshold effects. Indeed, different conclusions might be drawn even using sublines of the same cell line as is shown in Fig. 3 (Wallner et al. 1987). The data shown for HA-M3 cells (a mitomycin C resistant clone of HA-1) cast doubt on the existence of a "threshold" temperature. For another resistant clone, HA-M4, a threshold might be said to exist near 42 °C. For HA-1, a break occurs near 43 °C. In the case of the three platinum compounds, it actually appears that a relatively low threshold temperature exists for all three agents (sensitization appears above approximately 40.0 °C (see Cohen and Robins 1990b; Cohen et al. 1989a). Perhaps then, instead of considering drugs as either exhibiting or not exhibiting thresholds, it might be more accurate to simply view different drugs as having different threshold temperatures. These two hypotheses have not been formally tested.

The data in Fig. 8, showing that thermal enhancement can rapidly increase with small changes in temperature, highlight the importance of precise thermometry during WBH (Cohen and Robins 1990b). In addition, thermal sensitization does not necessarily just keep increasing with rising temperature. For instance, cisplatin (Fisher and Hahn 1982), carboplatin, and tetraplatin (Cohen and Robins 1990b) exhibit maximal enhancement at approximately 42 °C without further enhancement at higher temperatures (see Fig. 8).

4.3.3 Heating Duration

Conceivably, thermal enhancement might be different for two different heating durations. This possibility has been studied in many experimental systems. In at least one in vivo model it appears that the heating duration must be at least one half hour to have an apparent tumoricidal effect (Joiner et al. 1982). In vitro, as is shown in Fig. 9 (Cohen and Robins 1987), thermal sensitization is constant for multiple heating-drug durations from 0.5 to 3.5 h. In this experiment, the temperature and drug concentration were constant at 41.8 °C and 30 µg/ml respectively (Cohen and Robins 1987). Correction of survival (heat plus drug) for thermal killing (heat alone) yields a constant thermal enhancement effect for all time points. Thus, changing the duration of combined drug-WBH exposure should not affect the magnitude of the thermal enhancement effect but should alter the net cytotoxicity achieved (Cohen and Robins 1987). An early example of this same effect is shown in Fig. 10 for doxorubicin (Adriamycin) and 43 °C in HA-1 cells in vitro (Hahn and Strande 1976) where the sensitization effect remains relatively stable for up to 240 min.

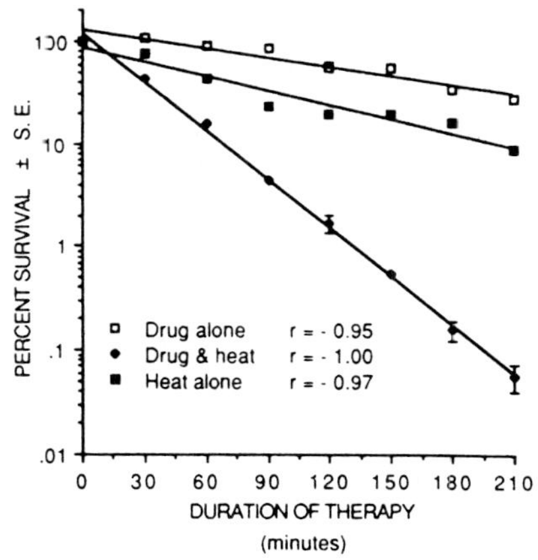

Fig. 9. Effect of treatment duration on survival. Cells were exposed to heat alone (41.8 °C), to carboplatin alone (30 µg/ml), or to carboplatin and heat simultaneously and then plated at 30-min intervals. The data for combined heat and carboplatin are not corrected for direct heat killing (Cohen and Robins 1987)

4.3.4 Thermal Tolerance

During WBH, it is conceivable that the time needed to reach target temperature might affect the degree of thermal chemosensitization. In particular, prolonged gradual heating en route to the target temperature might permit the development of thermal tolerance. It has been suggested that tumor cells, under such conditions, might not be as strongly sensitized by hyperthermia as with rapid heating (Herman et al. 1982a). Some observations (e.g., Herman et al. 1982a) have been compatible with such a scenario with a prolonged time to target temperature resulting in decreased thermal sensitization compared to cells placed immediately at the target temperature (the drug is added upon reaching target temperature). In other studies, induction of thermal tolerance has been associated with reduced thermal chemosensitization (Morgan et al. 1979).

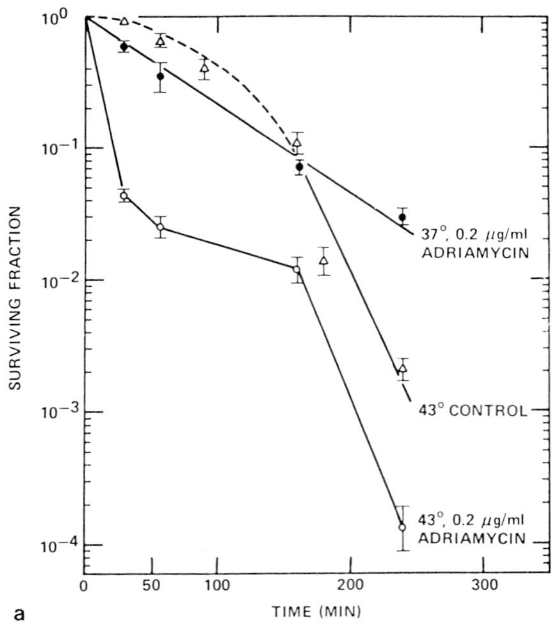

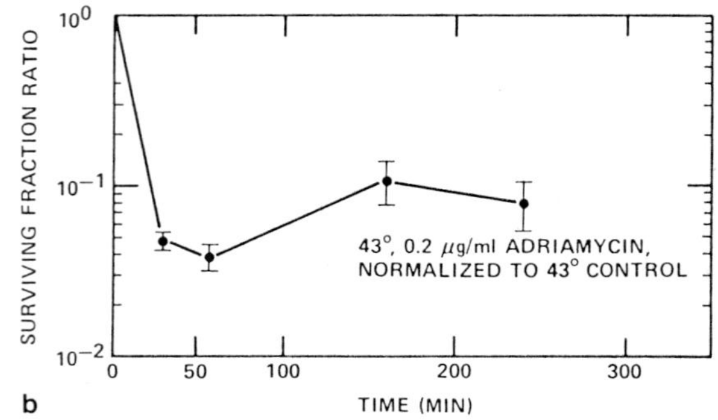

Fig. 10 a, b. Time response of HA-1 cells exposed simultaneously to 43 °C and Adriamycin. **a** Survival values. **b** Surviving fraction ratios which were obtained by dividing, point by point, the values of the lowest curve in **a** by the 43 °C control values. The *curve* is a measure of the cytotoxic action of Adriamycin at 43 °C (Hahn and Strande 1976)

We prefer a more direct approach to the question that such thermotolerance or heating duration studies really should be driving at – how, in fact, time to reach target temperature, heating duration, or the development of thermal tolerance affects the *therapeutic index* of WBH-drug therapy. Unfortunately, it is completely unknown how a prolonged time to target temperature or the development of thermal tolerance or variations in heating time might affect normal cells as opposed to tumor cells. In effect then, the only clinically important question about thermal tolerance has never been formally asked or studied. Clearly, factors such as thermal tolerance (if it occurs to a meaningful extent) could improve, worsen, or not even change the therapeutic index for a WBH-chemotherapy treatment regimen.

4.3.5 Decreased pH and pO_2

At least in vitro, thermal chemosensitization appears greater at lower pH for BCNU and bleomycin (Hahn and Shiu 1983) as is shown in Fig. 11 (Hahn and Shiu 1983). In the same studies, enhancement of amphote-

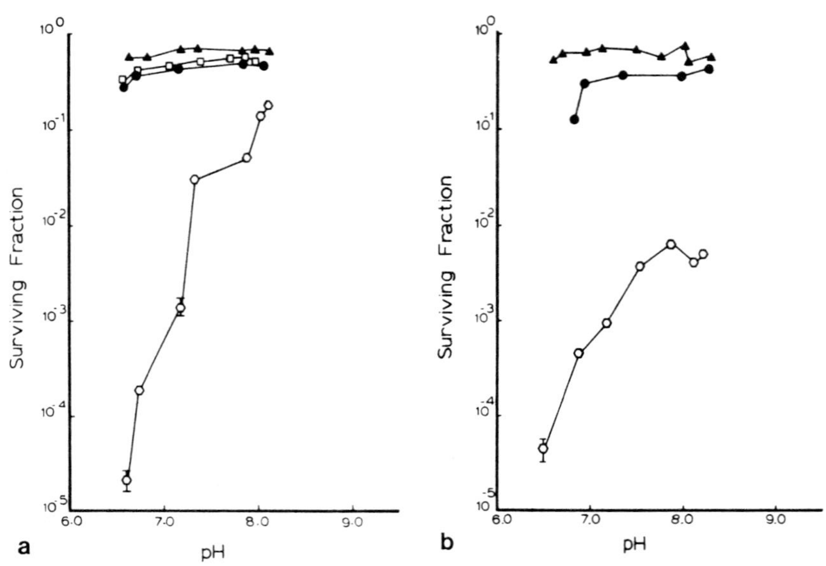

Fig. 11. a Influence of pH on the fraction of cells surviving BCNU treatment. ▲, 3.30 μg/ml at 37 °C for 1 h; □, 0.03% ethanol at 43 °C for 1 h; ●, 43 °C heat only; ○, 3.30 μg/ml at 43 °C for 1 h. *Bars*, SEM. **b** Influence of pH on survival of cells exposed to bleomycin treatment. ▲, 15 μg/ml at 37 °C for 1 h; ●, 43 °C heat only; ○, 15 μg/ml at 43 °C for 1 h. *Bars*, SEM (Hahn und Shiu 1983)

ricin B killing varied in a more complex manner with the least synergism at a pH of 7.4, i.e., the interaction was greater at higher or lower pH (Hahn and Shiu 1983). This effect is seen whether cells are acutely or chronically at low pH (Hahn and Shiu 1983, 1986) and might help to explain, for example, why thermal enhancement of BCNU killing may be greater in larger than in smaller tumors (Li and Hahn 1984). In vitro studies also suggest that hypoxic conditions enhance the cytotoxicity of doxorubicin, mitomycin C, and porfiromycin (Teicher et al. 1981a; Pritsos and Sartorelli 1986).

Perhaps the effects of hypoxia and reduced pH are both related to the increased thermal sensitivity of cells under such conditions. It is also possible that these effects could involve some common mechanisms since the dependence of hypoxic cells on anaerobic glycolysis may reduce pH intracellularly and in the local microenvironment.

One study combining cyclophosphamide and hyperthermia highlights the potential complexities of physiologic systems involved in heat-drug interactions in vivo. In this study, the authors considered evidence (Urano and Kim 1983) that (a) thermal enhancement of cyclophosphamide cytotoxicity correlates with the degree of thermal injury in several experimental systems, (b) thermal injury is greater at lower pH, and (c) hyperglycemia can reduce tumor tissue pH (perhaps selectively because of the preferential dependence on anaerobic glycolysis in some tumor cells) (Kim JH et al. 1978; Kim SH et al. 1978, 1980). Therefore, they predicted that glucose and hyperthermia together might produce greater enhancement of cyclophosphamide killing than would heat alone. As is shown in Fig. 12 (Urano and Kim 1983), *local* hyperthermia (41.5 °C for 90 min) with cyclophosphamide increased the median tumor growth time (until half of tumors reached 1000 mm^3) 1.31-fold compared to using cyclophosphamide alone (Urano and Kim 1983) (using the FSA-II spontaneous murine fibrosarcoma injected into footpads which were then heated by immersing in water baths). With glucose and heat together growth delay was 2.86-fold, substantially more than with heat alone. Glucose alone at 37 °C did not enhance cyclophosphamide growth inhibition (Urano and Kim 1983).

We find these results quite interesting. However, the exact degrees of cell killing are not evident from these types of experiments and it is not clear whether glucose primarily affected thermal killing or cyclophosphamide killing. It is also not entirely clear whether these results could apply to the use of cyclophosphamide with WBH or to the use of glucose with WBH thermochemotherapy. The effects of leg immersion

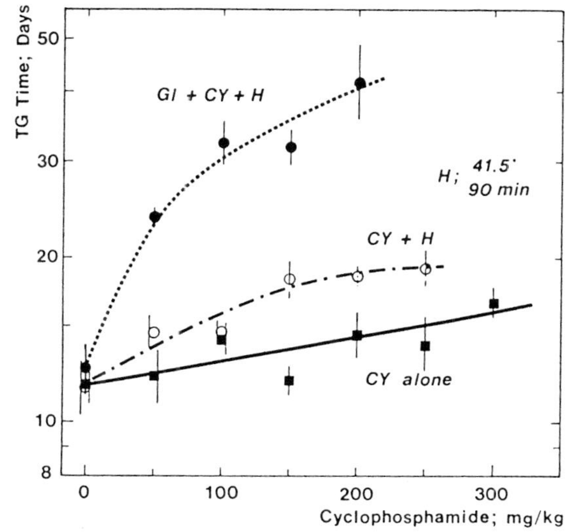

Fig. 12. Effect of hyperglycemia on thermochemotherapy. The FSA-II tumors were treated with cyclophosphamide (*CY*) alone, CY and hyperthermia (*H*), or glucose (*Gl*), CY, and heat. Hyperthermia was for 90 min at 41.5 °C, and the glucose dose was 10 mg/g. The tumor growth (TG) time was shown as a function of CY dose. *Bars*, 95% confidence limits (Urano and Kim 1983)

on core body temperature were not reported (Urano and Kim 1983) and it is quite possible that core body temperature rose only slightly or not at all. Obviously, changes in core body temperature could profoundly alter the metabolism of either glucose or of cyclophosphamide.

4.4 Therapeutic Index

Myelosuppression is the dose-limiting toxicity for many chemotherapeutic drugs. However, for some drugs other toxicities are prominent such as with cisplatin nephrotoxicity (Loehrer and Einhorn 1984) and acute or chronic doxorubicin cardiac toxicity. There is little information available regarding doxorubicin cardiotoxicity; i.e., it has been *suggested* that WBH and doxorubicin in combination might increase endogenous catecholamine release resulting in cardiac rhythm disturbances (Kim et al. 1979a, b). This possibility is based upon a single report involving one patient (water perfusion suit-WBH technology without prophylactic lidocaine) for whom very few catecholamine measurements are available and for whom only limited pretreatment cardiac studies were available. Based on this case report, caution is indicated if doxorubicin is to be a component of future WBH clinical trials. However, additional information is clearly needed, especially using other WBH technologies, before the existence and general relevance of this phenomenon can be accepted.

Some data also exist regarding the effects of WBH on doxorubicin metabolism and tissue distribution in rabbits (Mimnaugh et al. 1978). Rates of clearance of doxorubicin from plasma were similar in hyperthermic (42.3 °C rectally) and normothermic (39.7 °C rectally) rabbits except for slightly accelerated drug clearance in the alpha distributive phase as is shown in Fig. 13 (Mimnaugh et al. 1978). Also, tissue drug levels were significantly higher in skeletal muscle and in duodenum for hyperthermic animals. Perhaps the most interesting finding of this experiment was that tissue drug uptake was not significantly different between the two groups of animals for any other tissues. It is especially worth pointing out that cardiac muscle doxorubicin levels were 18% greater in heated animals than in controls but this difference was not statistically significant (Mimnaugh et al. 1978). Thus, for temperatures near 42 °C it would currently be difficult to attribute thermal enhancement of doxorubicin cardiotoxicity to increased drug uptake.

For cisplatin, rather solid data suggest that WBH does not improve and may even decrease the therapeutic index. Specifically, Wondergem et al. have shown that WBH increases nephrotoxicity to about the same extent as drug killing is increased (Wondergem et al. 1988). In humans, WBH resulted in severe life-threatening nephrotoxicity which was not seen with other drugs using the same WBH apparatus (Gerad et al. 1983).

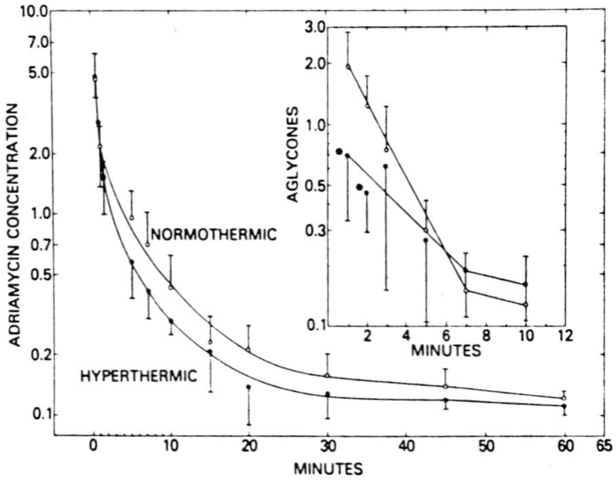

Fig. 13. The plasma concentrations of Adriamycin and total aglycones (μg/ml) in normothermic (○) and hyperthermic (●) rabbits following Adriamycin administration (5 mg/kg). The data are expressed as the means ±SD ($n = 5-7$). *, values that are significantly different from controls ($p < 0.05$) (Mimnaugh et al. 1978)

Very limited information is available regarding the effect of WBH on the therapeutic index of drugs which primarily cause myelosuppression. Preliminary evidence involving the treatment of AKR leukemia with carboplatin at 41.5 ° ±0.5 °C using radiant heat WBH suggests a therapeutic gain. Tumor survival decreased to an extent equivalent to a TER of 3.5 but myelosuppression was only minimally affected (Tapazoglou et al. 1988).

Honess and Bleehan showed a supraadditive interaction between 41 °C WBH (for 45 min) and BCNU or cyclophosphamide using spleen colony methodology with normal marrow stem cells and RIF-1 tumor in C3H/He mice (Honess and Bleehan 1982). There was no apparent therapeutic gain in this setting.

In very similar experiments, a therapeutic gain was suggested when using 41 °C WBH for 46 min and melphalan (Honess and Bleehan 1985a, b). Therapeutic ratios (the dose modifying factor for neoplastic cells divided by the dose modifying factor for normal cells) for melphalan were 1.9 – 2.0 for KHT sarcoma and 1.1 – 1.8 for RIF-1 fibrosarcoma grown in the hind legs of female C3H/He mice. These ratios were based on tumor growth delay (RIF-1 and KHT) and clonogenic cell survival (RIF-1 only) compared to spleen colony formation by normal marrow stem cells (Honess and Bleehan 1985b). Using smaller lung microtumors instead of the relatively larger limb tumors, therapeutic ratios for melphalan were lower for RIF-1 (0.8 – 1.4) and KHT (1.1 – 1.6), perhaps due to microvascular or nutritional factors (e.g., pH, hypoxia, etc.) (Honess and Bleehan 1985a).

These excellently conducted investigations by Honess and Bleehan highlight the formidable challenges which can be involved when assessing therapeutic index. Despite the considerable amount of work which was performed, it is not clear whether the findings for melphalan at 41 °C apply to (a) WBH at or near 41.8 °C, (b) to other cell lines, (c) to other WBH methodologies, or (d) to varying patterns/sequences of WBH and drug administration. In addition, it is not clear whether lung colony formation, spleen colony formation, tumor regrowth delay, etc. undergo equivalent changes in response to changes in treatment, i.e., the addition of WBH to the melphalan. Thus, it is conceivable that the observed therapeutic ratios could be survival assay artifacts which either underestimate or overestimate the therapeutic gain. Unfortunately, it is difficult to imagine a better way to conduct such studies except perhaps for the use of a single type of survival assay on closely related normal and neoplastic cell types, e.g., colony formation to assess both leukemic cell and normal bone marrow stem cell survival (e.g., Robins et al. 1984a).

4.5 Probable Thermal Sensitizing Agents

Table 4. Probable thermal sensitizing or labilizing compounds

Drug	In vitro studies	In vivo studies
Amphotericin B	+ (Hahn et al. 1977)	+ (Hahn and Li 1982)
S-(2-amino-ethyl)isothiouronium bormide		+ (Hahn 1979)
Ethanol	+ (Schrek and Stefani 1981)	+ (Anderson et al. 1983[a]; Hahn and Li 1982)
Lanthanum	+ (Marchal et al. 1986)	+ (Marchal et al. 1986)
Lidocaine	+ (Robins et al. 1984a)	+ (Yatvin 1977)
Lonidamine	+ (Kim JH et al. 1984b)	+ (Kim Jh et al. 1984b)
Misonidazole	+ (Morgan and Bleehan 1981b; Langer et al. 1982; Aaland et al. 1982)	+ (Lehman and Stewart 1983)
Quercetin	+ (Kim JH et al. 1984a)	

+, exhibiting thermal sensitizing effect.
[a] Heating was at 43.5 °C. Also, the mice were treated with pentobarbital, a potentially complicating factor (Anderson et al. 1983).

Table 4 lists agents which are "labilizers" or have been considered to exhibit a "thermal sensitizing" effect.

4.6 Future Directions for Preclinical Research

As we have discussed, only a few studies have attempted to precisely quantify whether WBH can produce a therapeutic gain in combination with various chemotherapeutic drugs. This lack of information is not surprising given the tedious and costly in vivo methods involved in precisely quantifying the relative survival of neoplastic cells and normal hematopoietic cells. Moreover, at this time, few laboratories are skilled in the administration of WBH to multiple experimental animals.

Nevertheless, in regard to the future progress of WBH and chemotherapy, it is reasonable to suggest that the greatest need today is to systematically clarify (a) for which drugs WBH might produce a therapeutic gain, and (b) the impacts of multiple potential treatment variables (temperature, heating duration, drug dosage, heat-drug sequence) on therapeutic index. The first step in addressing this need is simply to recognize that sizeable "blind spots" exist in this key area of knowledge.

4.7 Clinical WBH Studies

Clinical WBH-chemotherapy investigations have proceeded in three overlapping stages. First, a series of very early, small pilot studies was conducted. These investigations, based on relatively limited preclinical data, were designed primarily to test the practicality of combining new WBH methodologies with certain chemotherapy drugs. Next came a group of similar pilot studies which were based on much more abundant preclinical information. Finally, a third group of studies have formally addressed the types of questions that are typical of traditional phase I, II, and III clinical trials.

In discussing early small pilot studies, a good place to begin is with three clinical studies reported in 1979. One investigation reported by J. M. Larkin in 1979 involved 29 patients who were given 42.0 °C WBH (using a water blanket heating method) in combination with either 5-FU (9 mg/kg), cyclophosphamide (200 mg/m^2), or dacarbazine (DTIC) (200 mg/m^2). Overall, 59% of these patients were reported as having responses – although the distribution of responses by type of chemotherapy was not reported and the sequencing of the modalities is not clear. In comparison, there were responses in 52% of patients who received only WBH (Larkin 1979). This approach produced hyponatremia, hypokalemia, metabolic acidosis, hypocalcemia, hypomagnesemia, hypophosphatemia, probably disseminated intravascular coagulation, elevation of serum glutamic-oxaloacetic transaminase, lactate dehydrogenase, and creatine phosphokinase. Five deaths were attributed to WBH treatment (Larkin 1979).

In the same year, Parks and coworkers reported on a series of 25 patients with bronchogenic carcinomas (2 small cell and 23 nonsmall cell) who received 97 WBH treatments (41.5°–43.0 °C by arteriovenous (AV) shunt with extracorporeal heating) with cyclophosphamide (250 mg/m^2) and BCNU (50 mg) being given at the midpoint of the WBH. Occasional toxicities were thrombophlebitis with embolization (one patient), shunt infection (one patient), and rhabdomyolysis (one patient). Two deaths were attributed to the WBH. Generally observed toxicities or concerns included decreased platelet numbers without elevated fibrin split products, intrapulmonary shunting responsive to positive end expiratory pressure, and hypophosphatemia. Responses in this study included three complete responses and ten partial responses (Parks et al. 1979).

A third study published in 1979 was conducted by Barlogie and colleagues who treated 13 cancer patients with either 41.9 °C WBH alone (7 patients) or two treatments with WBH alone followed by a third treatment with WBH plus melphalan (5 patients), or etoposide (1 patient). Of the 11 patients who were evaluable for response, four had minor responses to WBH alone. Clinical toxicity in the 12 patients (one refused further treatment after two WBH sessions) included first-, second-, and third-degree burns (8, 5, and 1 patient respectively), herpes simplex eruptions (6 patients), posttreatment fevers, severe fatigue, diarrhea (6 patients), rhabdomyolysis (1 patient with WBH alone), four episodes of peripheral neuropathy, and two episodes of seizures. Laboratory abnormalities included marked neutropenia (several patients), hypocalcemia, hypomagnesemia, hypophosphatemia, elevated creatine phosphokinase (in all patients) as well as platelet count reduction, elevated prothrombin time and partial thromboplastin time with hypofibrogenemia in four patients. Unfortunately, in this report, toxicity due to combined modality therapy was generally not distinguished from toxicity due to WBH alone (Barlogie et al. 1979).

These three investigations illustrate the challenges and difficulties associated with the earliest clinical WBH studies. Moreover, although these studies were not designed to assess the frequency of responses, they did show that WBH plus chemotherapy produced at least some antitumor effect. Unfortunately, this positive aspect was overshadowed by the often severe morbidity and occasional mortality in these small WBH patient populations – a problem related to the WBH technologies being employed and to the patient selection criteria. In addition, *with the benefit of hindsight*, it is now apparent that some patients received drugs which one would not expect to interact with WBH in a supraadditive manner (e.g., etoposide, 5-FU, and probably cyclophosphamide). Moreover, WBH alone and the drugs by themselves have antineoplastic efficacy. Thus, it is not clear that the observed antitumor effects were due to WBH-drug interactions.

This pattern was repeated to varying extents over the next 6 years, i.e., provocatively frequent responses (of uncertain origin) with high morbidity. However, as is discussed earlier in this chapter, a wealth of preclinical data on heat-drug interactions and sequencing became available in the early 1980s permitting somewhat clearer drug selection and study design. For example, Herman et al. described 11 patients who received 30 WBH-chemotherapy treatments at temperatures of 42.0°, 42.2°, and 42.4 °C for 3 h ("depending on tolerance") with the treatments being given 7–10 days apart (Herman et al. 1982c). WBH was induced by heating blanket (six patients) or by extracorporeal heating (five patients). Upon reaching target temperature, four patients received intravenous cisplatin (60 mg/m^2) and four were given intravenous BCNU (50 mg/m^2). One patient receiving BCNU was also given methylGAG for 3 days prior to the WBH-BCNU treatment (Herman et al. 1982c).

Of the ten evaluable patients, six had partial responses which were very short lived, i.e., 5–24 weeks. Toxicity in this study included 2 treatment-related deaths, severe fatigue (all patients), neutropenia (3 treatments), thrombocytopenia (13 treatments), disseminated intravascular coagulation (10 treatments), peripheral neuropathy (1 treatment), seizures (1 treatment), hallucinations (1 treatment), cutaneous burns (5 patients), hemorrhage into pulmonary metastasis (1 treatment), hepatic necrosis in the absence of hepatic tumor (1 treatment), ventricular fibrillation (1 patient), ventricular tachycardia (1 other patient), leukopenia (3 treatments), and nearly all patients developed generalized anasarca including, in some patients, a pulmonary capillary leak syndrome. Other findings included marked hypotension, hypophosphatemia, hypocalcemia, hypomagnesemia, fluctuations in serum potassium, as well as elevated creatine phosphokinase, SGOT, and lactate dehydrogenase levels (Herman et al. 1982c). Unfortunately, the presence or absence of renal toxicity was not reported for the cisplatin-treated patients (Herman et al. 1982c). (The presence or absence of nephrotoxicity is of interest in relation to the subsequent report of clear-cut marked thermal enhancement of cisplatin nephrotoxicity [Gerad et al. 1983]. The study showing nephrotoxicity, which we have previously mentioned [Gerad et al. 1983], used a "space suit" methodology [see Bull et al. 1979a]. Interestingly, this WBH technique did not produce nephrotoxicity when used with other drugs [Gerad et al. 1983, 1984]).

In another small study, 13 patients received 16 WBH treatments at 40.5°–41.9 °C for 200–450 "degree min" with BCNU (50%–75% of the "normal" BCNU dose) at the midpoint of the hyperthermia plateau phase. At the highest treatment level (450 degree min and 75% BCNU dose), this regimen resulted in severe thrombocytopenia ($<10000/mm^3$) in three of three patients, two- to threefold prothrombin time elevation, "tremendous" liver function abnormalities, and a Guillain-Barré-like polyneuropathy in one patient (Selker et al. 1983).

One year later Gerad and coworkers reported a series of 11 patients with advanced soft tissue sarcomas (9 patients) or mesothelioma (2 patients) and no prior chemotherapy who received 41.8°–43.0 °C WBH (water perfusion suit) for 2 h in combination with doxorubicin and cyclophosphamiode (Gerad et al. 1984). These patients underwent initial chemotherapy courses at normal body temperature to permit baseline pharmacokinetic studies. This was followed by a total of 35 combined modality treatments in which doxorubicin (46 mg/m^2) was given at the beginning of the peak temperature and cyclophosphamide (1000 mg/m^2) was given 6 h later. This approach was associated with two complete responses, two partial responses, and two "disease stabilizations" (Gerad et al. 1984).

Once again, morbidity was considerable, the 11 patients experiencing reversible neuropathy (20% of treatments), hypotension, posttreatment electrolyte shifts (especially hypophosphatemia), cardiac arrhythmias (premature ventricular contractions or supraventricular tachycardia during 20% of treatments), fatigue and anasarca (100% of treatments), myalgias (20% of treatments), thrombocytopenia, hepatic enzyme elevation, nausea and vomiting (66% of treatments), diarrhea (9 of 11 patients), marked rises of skeletal muscle creatine phosphokinase (3 of 11 patients), posttreatment hypoglycemia (after one treatment), obtundation lasting 48 h (after one treatment), small first- or second-degree surface burns (37% of treatments), fever with granulocytopenia (3 of 11 patients), and perioral herpes simplex (8 of 11 patients) (Gerad et al. 1984).

In the same group of studies should be included the work of Koga and coworkers in Japan who in 1985 reported 17 patients with advanced gastrointestinal malignancies treated with 41.5°–42.0 °C WBH for 3–5 h (femoral arterial AV shunt with extracorporeal heating) with or without 1-(2-tetrahydrofuryl)-5-FU (tegafur) or 5-FU or mitomycin C with or without cyclophosphamide (Koga et al. 1985). All 17 patients were previously refractory to tegafur, 5-FU, or mitomycin C. Basically, a 3- to 5-h infusion of 5-FU (500–700 mg/m^2) with or without cyclophosphamide (100–200 mg/m^2) was started upon reaching the target temperature and an intravenous injection of mitomycin C (5–10 mg/m^2) was given at the midpoint of the heating course. After the WBH session patients then received mitomycin C (5–10 mg/m^2/week) and tegafur (300–400 mg/m^2/day) (Koga et al. 1985).

This approach resulted in partial responses in 2 of 12 patients with gastric cancer and in 1 of 5 patients with colon cancer equal to 23.1% of the 13 evaluable patients (4 patients died early in this population with advanced disease). Toxicity included lower extremity weakness which in some patients appeared to be of neuropathic origin (12 patients), thrombocytopenia (13 patients) including protracted thrombocytopenia (1 patient), leukocytopenia (8 patients), AV shunt infection (1 patient), AV shunt thrombosis (1 patient), intraabdominal bleeding (1 patient), hepatorenal syndrome (2 patients), and transient bilirubin and creatine phosphokinase elevation. Overall, four patient deaths were attributed to WBH with specific causes of death including intraabdominal bleeding (one patient), pulmonary edema (one patient), and hepatorenal syndrome (two patients). Each death involved patients with very advanced hepatic or renal disease (Koga et al. 1985).

This research group eventually completed a much larger study including 168 patients with miscellaneous advanced malignancies who received a total of 444 extracorporeally induced WBH treatments (Maeta et al. 1987). The patients in this study received a variety of chemotherapy regimens with the regimens being determined by each of the seven participating hospitals. The drugs included cisplatin (63 patients), doxorubicin (32 patients), mitomycin C (23 patients), nimustine HCl (4 patients), bleomycin (2 patients); 6 patients received no chemotherapy. These various treatments produced responses in 29.5% of 132 evaluable patients (Maeta et al. 1987).

Toxicity included pulmonary edema (15 patients), hepatic insufficiency (16 patients), hemorrhage of tumor (12 patients) or elsewhere (17 patients), cardiovascular shock (6 patients), renal insufficiency (8 patients), local infection (6 patients), and central (25 patients) or peripheral neurotoxicity (20 patients) (Maeta et al. 1987). Deaths related to treatment complications occurred in 24 patients. Unfortunately, although the authors comment on the occurrence of nephrotoxicity, they do not specifically indicate the exact experience of those patients who received cisplatin.

It is difficult to assess the clinical implications of this large study given the uncontrolled, varying drug selection as well as the frequent choice of drugs which are of questionable value in combination with WBH.

Overall this second group of clinical studies had some success in setting the stage for larger, formal phase I, II, and III investigations of WBH with chemotherapy. Unfortunately, at the same time, the frequent WBH-related morbidity and continued occasional mortality contributed to a deepening skepticism regarding the potential clinical utility of WBH-chemotherapy.

In very recent years a series of formal phase I, II, and even phase III clinical studies have been reported which have involved much more acceptable toxicities and more traditional experimental designs. For example, R. Engelhardt and colleagues have recently reported preliminary results on three disease-specific studies combining WBH and chemotherapy. These have dealt with small cell lung cancer, non-small-cell lung cancer, and malignant melanoma respectively (this group used a "Siemen's box" – a plexiglass chamber containing air heated to 55°–60 °C with patients resting on a mattress containing a coil field electrode connected to a 27-MHz generator).

The small cell lung carcinoma study was a prospective study involving patients with extensive stage disease who were randomized to receive six cycles of intravenous doxorubicin (60 mg/m^2 on day 1), oral cyclophosphamide (200 mg/m^2 on days 2–5), and intravenous vincristine (2 mg on day 1) either with or without day 1 hyperthermia (41° ± 0.5 °C for 1 h). To our knowledge, this is the only randomized, prospective clinical WBH investigation to date (Englehardt 1988). In this study, preliminary data were reported on 44 evaluable patients (out of 55) who were evenly divided between the two treatment groups. For the euthermic group the mean duration of response was 105 days (range 42–193), the mean leukocyte nadir was 3170/mm^3, and the mean platelet nadir was 231520/mm^3. For the hyperthermia group the mean duration of response was 130 days (range 53–392), the mean leukocyte nadir was 2440/mm^3 (significantly decreased, $p = 0.044$), and the mean platelet nadir was 169030/mm^3 (Englehardt 1988). The response rates and survival durations in this study do not compare well with results from some other small cell carcinoma trials which used chemotherapy without WBH (Minna et al. 1989). This may reflect the fact that the drug doses and dose intensity for this trial, which were chosen many years ago, were considerably lower than doses which have subsequently been shown to be optimal for small cell carcinoma (Minna et al. 1989). These concerns notwithstanding, this study is interesting in that WBH modestly improved the response duration suggesting either some drug-WBH interaction the therapeutic or an additive effect of the two modalities (it is not clear whether the therapeutic index was affected as WBH also modestly increased myelosuppression). It is also interesting to speculate as to what might have been observed using 41.8 °C instead of 40°–41.0 °C, larger patient numbers, or other drug combinations – especially given that only the doxorubicin should have been expected to have interacted with the hyperthermia.

In the nonsmall cell lung carcinoma trial, patients received cisplatin (100 mg/m^2 i.v. on day 1), vindesine (3 mg/m^2 i.v. on day 1), and etoposide (120 mg/m^2 i.v. on days 2 and 3). Hyperthermia was given on day 1. Day 1 drugs were injected upon reaching target temperature which was then maintained for 1 h (Englehardt 1988).

For this study, 14 patients have been described of which 7 were evaluable for response having completed two or more treatments. Thus, this study is too small to permit meaningful assessments of response rates. Nevertheless, among these seven patients there was one complete response and two partial responses (plus two minor responses). Toxicity included elevation of creatinine to 2.3 mg/ml, leukocyte counts below 3000/mm^3 in 9 of 18 treatment cycles and below 1000/mm^3 in 2 of 18 cycles; thrombocytopenia < 100000/mm^3 occurred in 2 of 18 cycles (Englehardt 1988).

In the similarly small pilot study dealing with malignant melanoma, 23 patients received cisplatin (80 mg/m^2 i.v. on day 1) with WBH (41 °C for 1 h), and doxorubicin (50 mg/m^2 i.v. on day 2), more than 24 h after WBH. The cisplatin was given when core body temperature reached 40.5 °C with the temperature then being held at 41 °C for 45–60 min. Out of 15 patients who were evaluable for response, there were 3 partial responses and 4 minor responses. Toxicity included leukocyte counts below 3000/mm^3 in 13 of 31 treatment cycles and below 2000/mm^3 in 5 of 31 cycles; thrombocytopenia under 100000/mm^3 occurred in 4 cycles (Englehardt 1988; Englehardt et al. 1990). Based on these results, the authors concluded that WBH with cisplatin resulted in response rates and drug toxicity comparable to data previously reported in the nonhyperthermia literature (Englehardt et al. 1990).

Certain aspects of the melanoma study make it difficult to accept this conclusion with absolute confidence. For example, the study was not a phase III study and contained too few patients to make such comparisons. More importantly, it is curious that WBH did not enhance cisplatin nephrotoxicity in these patients although such enhancement has clearly been observed in preclinical in vivo experimental systems (Wondergem et al. 1988) as well as in the clinical setting (Gerad et al. 1983). Conceivably, the lack of nephrotoxicity may relate to cisplatin administration when patients had barely reached 40.5 °C as well as to the relatively low target temperature of 41.0 °C. Is the lack of increased nephrotoxicity a hint that the heat-drug sequence or temperature were less than optimal with regard to thermal enhancement of cisplatin cytotoxicity? Actually, there is some suggestion that this could be the case; i.e., thermal enhancement of cisplatin, carboplatin, and tetraplatin cytotoxicity in vitro varies strongly with temperature (see Fig. 8) so that the use of 41 °C is a source for concern. Also, there is strong evidence that hyperthermia even immediately after platinum exposure yields little or no thermal chemosensitization (Cohen and Robins 1987; Corry et al. 1984; Wallner et al. 1986; Wallner and Li 1987). Thus, given the lack of pharmacokinetic data regarding the rate of drug distribution, the administration of cisplatin upon reaching only 40.5 °C raises the possibility that only a modest, difficult to detect sensitization effect could ever have been achieved in these patients.

Another recent clinical trial was the phase I assessment of radiant heat WBH with lonidamine (Robins et al. 1988a). In this study patients received excalating lonidamine doses of 60, 180, or 360 mg/m^2 orally per day (groups A, B, and C). The induction period consisted of WBH alone (41.0 °C for 85 min) on day 1, initiation of lonidamine on day 3 (continued throughout the remainder of treatment), one WBH treatment (41.0 °C for 85 min) during week 2, and two WBH treatments (41.8 °C for 85 min) in week 3. In the absence of progressive disease, patients then underwent one 41.8 °C WBH treatment during week 6, and two 41.8 °C WBH treatments in week 7. Patients with stable or responding disease then remained on lonidamine plus two 41.8 °C WBH sessions every 3–5 weeks (Robins et al. 1988a).

Overall, there were 93 WBH treatments at 41.0 °C and 105 WBH treatments at 41.8 °C. There were no responses in group A (3 patients), two partial responses and one improvement in group B (3 patients), and one complete response and two improvements in group C (17 patients) (Robins et al. 1988a). It is worth noting that one patient with nodular lymphoma responded to 180 mg lonidamine/m^2 in combination with 41.8 °C hyperthermia but not to the same lonidamine dose by itself or with 41.0 °C hyperthermia. The same patient also did not respond to 41.8 °C with 60 mg lonidamine/m^2. Thus, at least for this patient, the higher lonidamine dose and the higher temperature were both necessary to produce significant cytotoxic activity (Robins et al. 1988a).

Side effects potentially related to WBH included fatigue and lethargy lasting 24–48 h (5 of 23 patients), headaches during the first 6 h after WBH (5 patients), vomiting with minimal nausea (approximately 3 h after WBH due to thiopental gastric stasis in 5 patients), transient post-WBH fevers (3 patients), self-limited post-WBH herpes simplex of the lips (7 patients), post-WBH hiccups (1 patient), minor heel discomfort (2 patients), asymptomatic post-WBH hypovolemic hypotension (7 episodes promptly responsive to fluid administration), urinary tract infection (2 female patients), and calf thrombophlebitis (1 patient). Toxicities due to lonidamine, such as myalgias, testicular pain, photophobia, anorexia, and urinary frequency, were not increased by the addition of WBH (Robins et al. 1988a).

Finally, preliminary results have been reported regarding the combination of radiant heat WBH and carboplatin (Robins et al. 1990b). To date, six groups of three patients have received carboplatin doses of 100, 150, 200, 250, 300, and 350 mg/m^2 and are now being treated at 400 mg/m^2. So far, at the level of 350 mg carboplatin/m^2, WBH has not affected carboplatin myelosuppression and responses have occurred at carboplatin doses which are generally considered subtherapeutic (Calvert et al. 1982) at normal body temperature (e.g., 200 mg/m^2).

Collectively, this third group of studies has demonstrated the ability to combine chemotherapeutic drugs and WBH with acceptable WBH toxicity. Also, these studies have finally begun to provide formal estimates of toxicity and response frequencies. The one phase III study also offers very suggestive (but not definitive) evidence of supraadditive WBH-doxorubicin interaction in the clinical setting consistent with findings in the preclinical literature.

In considering the examples of clinical WBH-chemotherapy investigations that we have discussed as well as general principles of clinical research, it is possible to make several recommendations in regard to future clinical WBH-chemotherapy studies. First, the design of all future investigations must be based on rigorous statistical methods so as to include sufficient numbers of patients (and proper patient stratification) to permit clear answers to the clinical questions being posed in each study. When possible, phase I studies should be designed to compare pharmacokinetic and toxicological effects of drug alone, WBH alone, and drug plus WBH. Phase I studies should also involve only those drugs for which abundant preclinical data demonstrate thermal chemosensitization and, hopefully, some suggestion of therapeutic gain upon adding WBH (to some extent, therapeutic gain depends on the projected clinical setting, e.g., autologous BMT poses its own specific set of considerations). It is clear that phase II studies are needed to define those tumor types in which WBH might make a meaningful contribution. Given the variability between different cell lines and tumor types in preclinical studies, it will be necessary to clinically assess a variety of "promising" tumor types before drawing conclusions about the potential clinical utility of a given WBH-drug combination. These phase II studies should be based on preliminary assessments of maximally tolerated heat-drug doses from carefully conducted phase I studies. Rough dosage estimations based on preclinical data are not acceptable. Finally, it would be ideal if phase

III studies would await the results of well-conducted phase II trials. Only by adopting such a methodical, sequential approach (i.e., laboratory, phase I, phase II, and then phase III studies) can the true clinical utility of WBH chemosensitization be clearly determined.

5 Clinical and Biophysical Aspects of Systemic Hyperthermia

5.1 Thermal Regulation and WBH Methodologies

5.1.1 Review

If one excludes the induction of endogenous fevers by exogenous toxins or drugs, then all methodologies for WBH are dependent on the deposition of exogenous heat with supplementation of metabolic heat. In order to efficiently induce WBH, evaporative heat losses must be minimized. This can be easily accomplished by covering a patient so that an effective vapor barrier is created, or by producing a water-saturated atmosphere, e.g., with a humidification device.

Methodologies (see Fig. 1) for producing externally applied heat (reviewed in Table 1) include: immersion in hot wax or water; enclosure in heated water blankets or suits; exposure to hot air; exposure to radiant heat; the application of microwave energy, or diather-

Table 1. WBH technologies

Method	Temperature (°C)	Period of treatment (h)	Anesthesia/sedation	Reference
Bacterial toxin	~41		None	Coley 1893
Diathermy-radiant heat	41 – 41.5	5 – 21	NS	Warren 1935
Hot wax bath	41 – 41.8	2 – 4	Barbiturate, curare Epidural	Pettigrew et al. 1974a, b Levin and Blair 1978, 1982
Hot water blanket[a]	42	2 – 4	N_2O	Larkin et al. 1977; Larkin 1979
			N_2O, droperidol, fentanyl	Barlogie et al. 1979
			Barbiturate narcotics, fentanyl	Herman et al. 1982a, b
Extracorporeal	41.5 – 42	1 – 6	Thiopental, morphine, Valium, N_2O, Pavulon	Parks et al. 1979; Parks and Smith 1983
Water suit	39.5 – 41.8	1 – 4	Thiopental, fenttanyl	Bull et al. 1979a; Ostrow et al. 1981
Water suit (modified to include heated clinitron bed and general anesthesia)	39.5 – 41.8	1 – 4	N_2O, fentanyl, muscle relaxants	Cronau et al. 1984
Siemens box (hot air and microwave)	40 – 42	1	NS	Pomp 1978
	40 – 41	1	None	Neuman et al. 1982
Modified Siemens box (hot air and hot water blanket)	41.8 – 42	2	N_2O, methohexitone muscle relaxants	Van der Zee et al. 1983
Radiant heat	40.5 – 41.8	1 – 2.5	Thiopental, lidocaine, fentanyl, Valium	Robins et al. 1985b

NS, not stated.

[a] A variant of this approach is a hot water bath (Versteegh et al. 1981; Loshek et al. 1981; Selker et al. 1983).

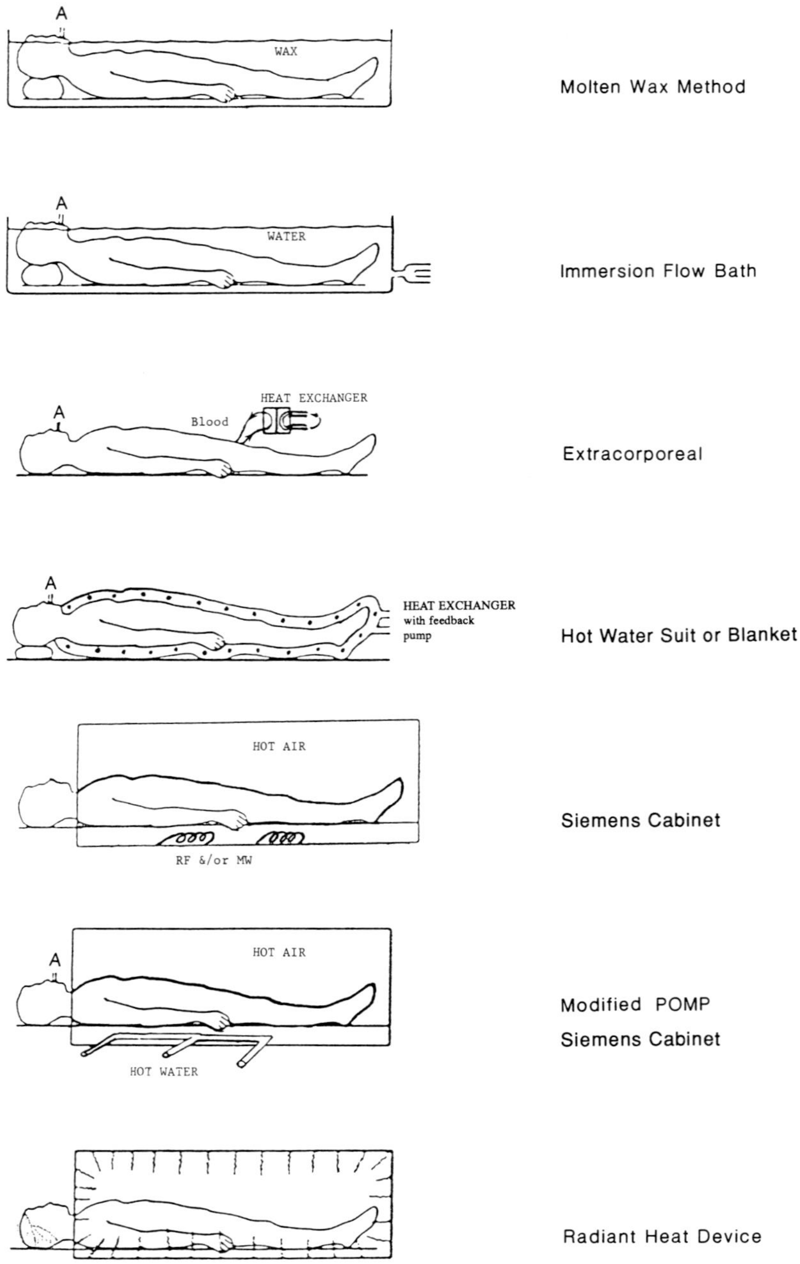

Fig. 1. WBH devices. *A*, general anesthesia; *RF*, radiofrequency (27 mHz); *MW*, microwave (433 – 468 mHz). (Modified after Van der Zee et al. 1987, 1990)

my – to a large area of the body. Beyond this, extracorporeal heating developed by Parks et al. (1979) involving the placement of a femoral AV shunt for the removal and replacement of blood (which is passed through a heat exchanger) represents the only other major technological approach to WBH. (It is of interest to note that peritoneal irrigation has also been used to produce 42 °C WBH [Priesching 1976].) For the reader's convenience, Table I partially summarizes the literature with regard to different WBH methodologies.

We and others have previously reviewed the essential aspects of thermal regulation as it relates to systemic hyperthermia in a series of manuscripts (Robins and Dennis 1981; Corry and Frazier 1982; Robins 1984, 1988; Robins et al. 1983b, d, 1985a, b; Robins and Neville 1986; Millgan 1984; Van der Zee et al. 1987, 1990).

In order to control and maintain target core temperatures many investigators have relied on computerized feedback loops (Bull et al. 1979a; Barlogie et al. 1979; Larkin 1979; Schuette et al. 1980). This approach, however, is not entirely necessary if the physiological changes which occur during WBH are exploited. As the core temperature of a human (or a large mammal – as will be reviewed later) increases there is a nonlinear increase in metabolic rate. This phenomenon is described (Law and Pettigrew 1980; Keele and Neil 1971) by the equation:

$$BMR_{Tcore} = \frac{85 \times 1.07^{(Tcore)}}{0.5},$$

This relationship is graphically illustrated in Fig. 2. When a patient is heated from 37 °C to a target core temperature of 41.8 °–42 °C, metabolic rate in a 70 kg man will have approximately doubled from 84 to 162 w. Thus, from the above discussion it should be recognized that metabolic heat is a key component of every WBH system. As we have previously discussed in detail (Robins et al. 1983 b, 1985 a, b), radiant heat losses, respiratory losses, and insensible losses at room temperature (when no significant evaporative losses are occurring) are the major factors in maintaining a human at normal body temperatures: the 84 w of basal metabolic heat produced by a human at room temperature are displaced to the environment by losses, i.e., respiration (−8 w), radiant heat (−48 w), and insensible losses (−29 w). At 41.8 °C core temperature, radiant heat losses become significantly greater, i.e., −107 w, due to an increase in skin temperature from 33 °C (at 37 °C core) to 39 °–40 °C (at 41.8 °C core); respiration losses (−8 w) and insensible losses (−29 w) are essentially unchanged at 41.8 °C compared to 37 °C. Thus, considering an increase in metabolic work to 162 w, simple addition demonstrates that a steady state of WBH can be maintained for several hours in the absence of evaporative heat losses. This steady state of WBH, sometimes referred to as the "plateau phase", can be ended when evaporative heat losses are permitted. To maintain temperatures significantly below 41.8 °C may require gentle supplementation with external heat to enter an appropriate equilibrium state.

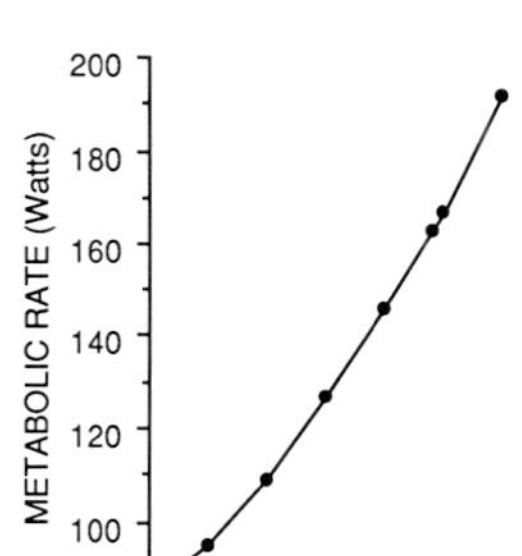

Fig. 2. The nonlinear relationship between increasing core temperature and metabolic rate

One important caveat to the above discussion relates to the danger of going above 42 °C with any WBH system. The nonlinear increase in metabolic rate which occurs with increasing core temperature makes thermal control fragile. Above 42 °C thermal compensatory mechanisms are already maximal, assuming that evaporative heat losses are minimal. Thus, a patient could enter a "thermal runaway" state due to what is essentially a self-perpetuating metabolic heat pump. This situation is in sharp distinction to malignant hyperthermia, a genetic disease described in man and pigs which is characterized by fever, muscle rigidity, and cardiac collapse after exposure to stress our drugs (Galant and Ahern 1983; Nelson and Flewellen 1983; Bell et al. 1983). Parenthetically, in our experience with pigs, a species which is far more physiologically "brittle" than humans during WBH, there was no hypothalamic thermoregulatory dysfunction after repeated exposure to ≥42 °C (Robins et al. 1983). This point is emphasized to highlight the concept that control mechanisms are saturated, not disabled.

5.1.2 WBH with a Regional Heat Boost

The above considerations are relevant to a proposal which is now receiving significant attention among different investigators: to perform WBH at a modest core temperature, e.g., ~41 °C and do a local-regional boost to a specific locus. If one deposits a significant amount of energy in the course of doing a local-regional boost during WBH, the deposited energy is quickly dissipated and the net result is to increase metabolic rate with a resultant increase in core temperature. This concept is graphically illustrated in Fig. 3, derived from our reported experience in performing radiant heat WBH with a microwave boost (Robins et al. 1983 c). We found that if exposure to microwave energy was significant and evaporative losses were not induced, core temperature increased; only if active cooling was allowed (through evaporative heat losses in this experiment) could a positive differential effect be achieved between core and local temperature. This experience was later observed in a canine model (Thrall et al. 1989 b, 1990). It is our current prejudice that the physiological complexities at play in performing WBH with a regional boost create a methodological scenario which requires an inordinate amount of effort to produce differences in regional temperatures. These differences will ultimately be modest at best.

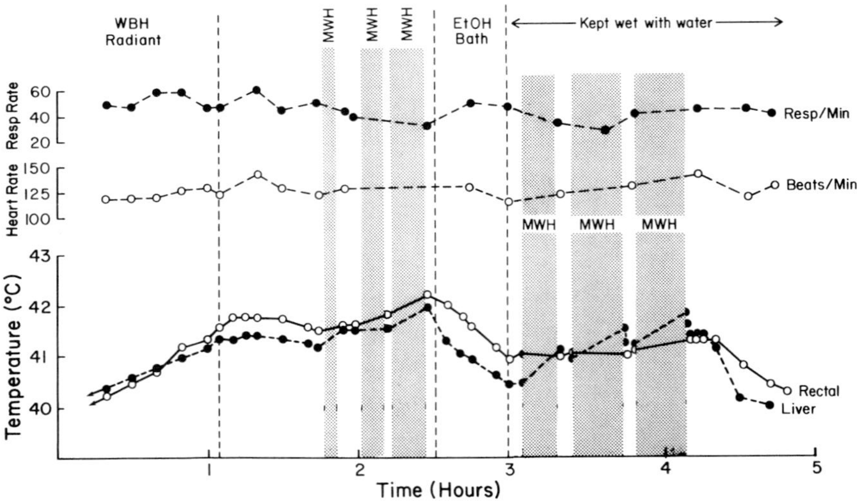

Fig. 3. WBH delivered with WBH-radiant heat device (RHD) microwave heat boost (*MWH*). MWH represented by *shaded area*. Note: period of radiant heat terminates at ~65 min. An alcohol bath is used to cool the animal prior to the commencement of the second phase of the first experiment. Following cooling with alcohol to a rectal temperature of 41 °C (in the first phase of the experiment) the pig received three additional MWH boosts. Throughout the period, i.e., the second phase of the experiment, the pig was kept wet with water to allow for continuing evaporative losses. EtOH, ethanol (Robins et al. 1983b)

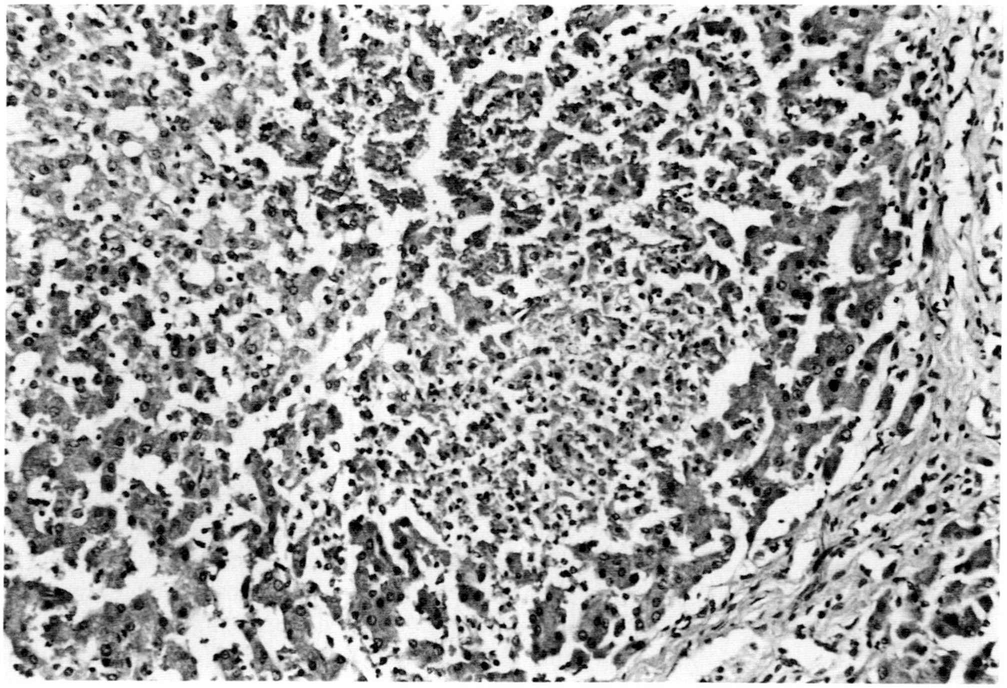

Fig. 4. Central hepatic necrosis after WBH with a regional boost using a porcine animal model

5.1.3 Electromagnetic Technology and WBH

The preclinical experience described above in addition to illustrating physiological principles and evaluating a concept, highlights the potential for accomplishing WBH with any of the currently acceptable regional electromagnetic hyperthermia technologies by simply minimizing evaporative heat losses. Indeed, at the University of Arizona such an approach is currently being explored (Shimm et al. 1989; Harari et al. 1990).

Although feasible, the deposition of large amounts of microwave energy to produce WBH is potentially compromised by unique problems not inherent in many other WBH systems which include: uneven deposition of energy during the heating phase – possibly causing tissue necrosis, unreproducible heating sessions, as well as thermometry and cardiac monitoring problems.

In this regard, Fig. 4 demonstrates a previously unpublished photomicrograph demonstrating central hepatic necrosis in a pig treated with regional WBH microwave hyperthermia. The limited (two probes) temperature monitoring done when the animal was treated did not suggest a liver temperature in excess of 42 °C. Thus, what was in retrospect believed to be an uneven heating session produced a significant toxicity. Full details describing the conditions of this experiment have been previously reported (Robins et al. 1983 b). Whether this porcine experience is relevant to clinical attempts to utilize microwave technology for WBH must be further defined in ongoing clinical research.

5.1.4 Summary

All species exchange heat by radiation, conduction, and convection. An understanding of this concept is essential to approaching the physiology of WBH. Recently, Schonbaum and Lomax (1990) edited a text which reviews a variety of subjects which may be of interest including thermal afferents in control of body temperature, functional mechanisms of temperature regulation, and neuropharmacological aspects of thermoregulation. Beyond this the reader may also wish to review a text by Houdas and Ring (1982) (which offers an excellent review of quantitative aspects of thermoregulation) as well as a classic paper by Cabanac (1975).

5.2 Monitoring Body Site Temperatures During WBH

As can be derived from the above discussion regarding the relationship of core temperature and metabolic rate, accurate continuous temperature monitoring is a requisite during WBH. This is particularly true when one is monitoring patients above 41 °C, when critical changes can occur in minutes; above 41.8 °C critical changes can occur in seconds!

It is our position, therefore, that in order to foresee trends in the final stages of the heating phase of WBH, temperature should be monitored to 0.01-degrees rather than 0.1-degrees accuracy as is the case with local and regional hyperthermia. Such precision not only results in greater patient safety, but also practically results in an increased uniformity of time-temperature profiles between treatments involving the same or different patients.

Additionally, patients should be monitored at multiple sites as will be described, since thermometry failure using only a single site can result in a lethal event (Pettigrew et al. 1974 b).

Most commercially available thermometry systems have accuracies of ~0.3 °–0.4 °C. Further, thermistors and thermocouples will demonstrate drifting over time. Thus, it is clear that any WBH program, which has as its goal core temperatures of 41.8 ° ±0.2 °C, should have a rigorous, formalized calibration protocol to check the accuracy and drift of thermometry. This is essential to ensure safe treatments. Additionally, toxicity and response data are extremely difficult to evaluate unless a research group has such a calibration program prospectively in place.

In general two approaches to WBH thermometry have been used, i.e., thermocouples and thermistors. The use of thermocouples for temperature monitoring is predicated on the use of two conductors (mode of different metals). The differences in voltage measured across the two conductors will vary as a function of temperature, i.e., the Seebeck effect. Unfortunately the relationship between temperature and changes in thermocouple voltage is nonlinear. Thermocouples tend to have a stable calibration curve as a function of time, but are less accurate than thermistors.

Thermistors in contrast, although more accurate than thermocouples, require recalibration frequently as they will change as a function of time. Thermistor use for thermometry is based on the inverse relationship between temperature and the resistance of a semiconductor. The sensitivity and accuracy of thermistors are excellent. It is noteworthy that when thermistors are calibrated, the calibration curve is specific for each thermistor, i.e., each thermistor being used must be individually calibrated.

We have preferred the use of thermistors for standard temperature monitoring, e.g., esophageal, rectal, skin – and the use of thermocouples for specialized invasive thermometry requiring thin probes, e.g., for tumor temperature measurements. For calibrations we have relied on a platinum resistance thermometer (Robins et al. 1985 b). The platinum-based systems as reference points are desirable, as the resistance of platinum is linear with temperature; these systems have a great deal of precision (+ or −0.02 °C) and have a high degree of long-term stability.

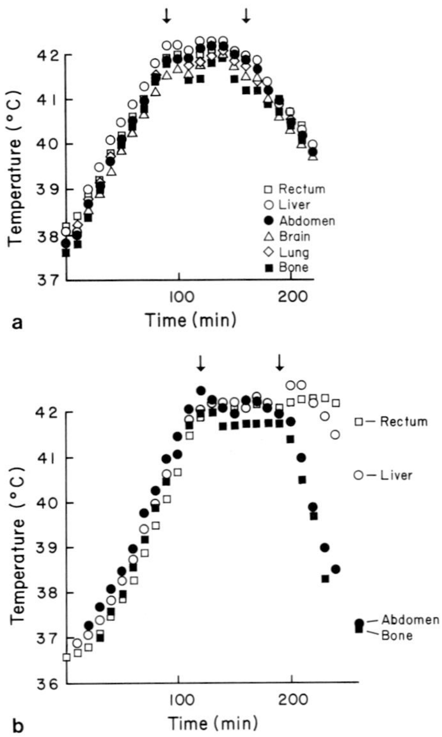

Fig. 5 a, b. Time-temperature profiles for various temperatures for two different dogs undergoing radiant heat WBH. The *first arrow* in **a** indicates the time that the animal reached 42 °C. The *second arrow* indicates the end of heating and beginning of active cooling. This dog received pentobarbital for anesthesia 25 mg/kg induction and 9 mg/kg per hour maintenance. The skin temperature during the hyperthermia plateau phase, i.e., time between the two arrows, was 41.10 °±0.39 °C ($n = 14$) for one probe and 40.11 °±0.39 °C ($n = 14$) for another prove. In **b** the *first arrow* indicates target temperature and the *second arrow* indicates the time at which the animal was sacrificed. The dog in **b** received 25 mg/kg pentobarbital for induction followed by 16.7 mg/kg per hour for maintenance. The skin temperature during the hyperthermia plateau phase, i.e., time between the two arrows, was 40.62 °±0.28 °C ($n = 16$) for one probe and 39.84 °±0.39 °C ($n = 15$) for another probe (Hugander et al. 1987)

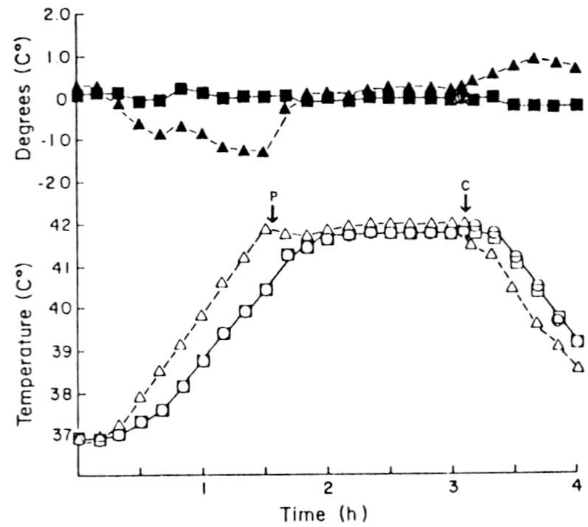

Fig. 6. *Lower panel* represents rectal (□), bladder (○), and esophageal (△) temperatures (T°) as a function of time. *Upper panel* presents the differences (T° bladder versus T° rectal, [■]; T° bladder versus T° esophageal, [▲]) in °C as a function of time. The *arrow P* indicates the patient achieving peak (target) temperature. At this time, the patient is covered with a vapor barrier. The *arrow C* indicates when the vapor barrier is removed and cooling of the patient begins (Martin et al. 1987)

It is necessary for the practltioner of WBH to understand the interrelationship of the temperature of various body sites during the heating phase, plateau phase, and cooling phase of WBH. One of the significant advantages of WBH over local and regional hyperthermia is the reproducibility of time-temperature profiles between treatments for a given subject, as well as the relative homogeneity of temperature for deep body sites during hyperthermia. This should be expected, particularly at plateau phase, as external heating is minimally required. Thus, metabolic heat, which is principally derived from the liver and brain; is constantly being redistributed through the body of any given subject. If a circulatory arrest is induced in a dog during WBH, liver and brain temperature is initially seen to increase – while decreasing in other tissues, consistent with these organs being dominant sources of metabolic heat (Hugander et al. 1987). This process is particularly effective as cardiac output (discussed in Sect. 5.3) is essentially double at ~41.8 °C core temperature during WBH. Fig. 5 illustrate various organ temperatures in a dog undergoing WBH.

Satisfactory estimates of arterial blood temperature can be obtained by an esophageal temperature probe (Dickson et al. 1979; Robins et al. 1985 b). The esophageal probe must be placed at the level of the heart in proximity to the great vessels. Despite the cautionary note of Parks and Smith (1983) regarding the importance of esophageal probe placement, we have found its use to be extremely reliable and accurate in everyday practice. The investigator who finds that esophageal temperature before treatment is reading below rectal temperature, merely needs to advance the probe slightly until there is agreement. The agreement between esophageal temperature and pulmonary artery temperature after proper positioning is invariably very good (Bull et al. 1979 a; Robins et al. 1985). We have further found that during the heating phase of WBH, a skin temperature probe placed over the axillary artery by first palpating this pulse, coupled with insulation taped over the probe, is an excellent approximation of esophageal and pulmonary ar-

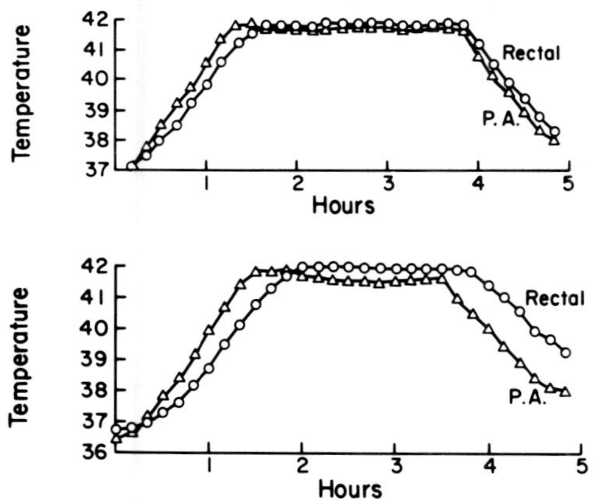

Fig. 7. The relationship of blood temperature (pulmonary artery, *PA*) to rectal temperature during the heating, plateau, and cooling phase of systemic hyperthermia performed, using two different patients, with an external heat system (Modified after Robins et al. 1985b)

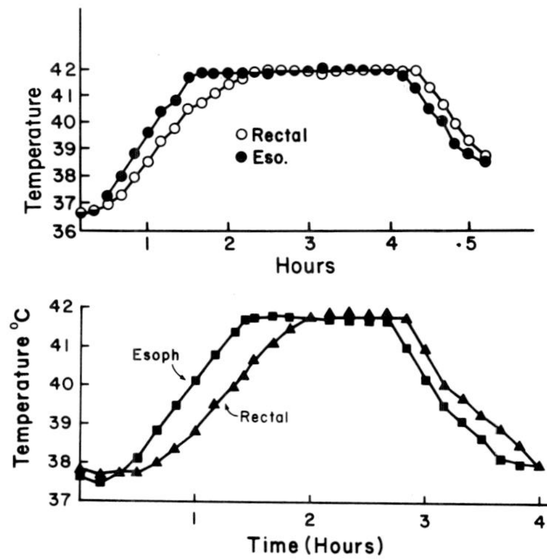

Fig. 8. The relationship of esophageal (○) temperature to rectal (●) temperature for a patient undergoing systemic hyperthermia with an external heating device (Modified after Robins et al. 1985a)

tery temperature during the heating phase of WBH. This axillary probe is less reliable during the plateau and cooling phase of WBH. Bladder temperature as measured by urinary bladder thermistor catheters has been proposed to measure blood temperature (Lilly et al. 1980). In a careful prospective WBH study, Martin et al. (1987) demonstrated that this is not the case. Such bladder probes actually reflect deep body temperature, e.g., rectal temperature (see Fig. 6). Tympanic membrane temperature can reflect blood temperature (Dickson et al. 1979). However, the use of tympanic membrane temperature probes is extremely placement sensitive; they can also easily move during treatment. We therefore discourage their use as part of a standard monitoring procedure.

As is logically expected, the temperatures of deep-seated body sites lag behind blood temperature during the heating phase of WBH. If heat is externally applied to the surface of the body, then skin temperature will run higher than core temperature (organ or blood) during the heating phase. During the plateau phase there is an equilibrium between blood and deep-seated organs. During this phase there will also be a rapid fall in the temperatures of skin or subcutaneous tissue as heat is being dissipated by radiant heat losses as discussed above. Finally, during the cooling phase of a treatment, blood temperature decreases before organ temperature decreases.

In order to familiarize the reader with the interrelationship between body sites (as well as between species), we have selected a series of figures from the literature demonstrating various time-temperature profiles obtained during WBH at different tissue sites. Figure 7 illustrates the relationship of pulmonary ar-

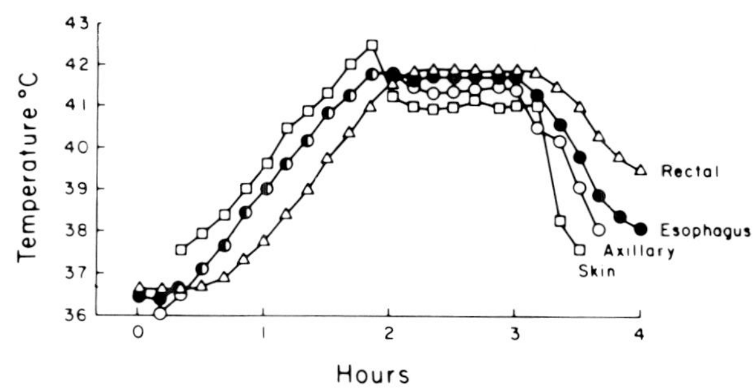

Fig. 9. The relationship of rectal, esophageal, axillary and skin temperature during radiant heat systemic hyperthermia (Modified after Robins et al. 1990a)

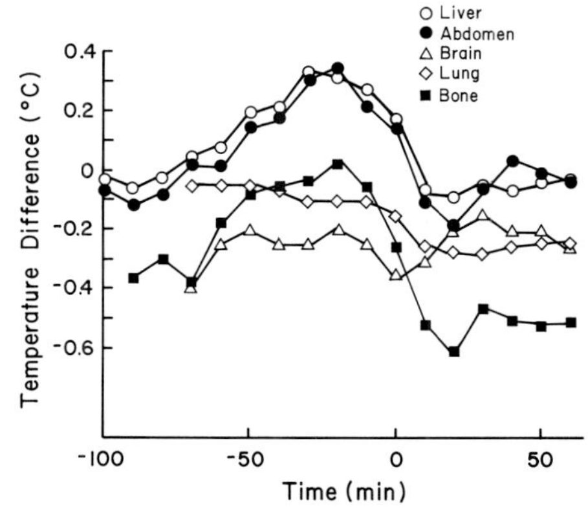

Fig. 10. Temperature distribution during WBH. Average difference ($n = 5$) between rectal temperature and various other sites (>0 indicates temperature exceeding rectal temperature). Before averaging, time was adjusted for all animals such that time zero was the time that the animal's rectal temperature reached the target temperature (Hugander et al. 1987)

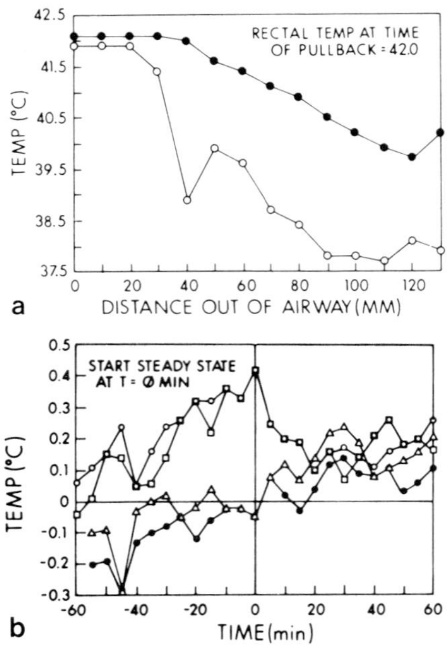

Fig. 11. a Lung temperature as a function of distance out of the airway in one dog undergoing WBH. ●, T_{max}; ○, T_{min}. **b** Brain temperature minus rectal temperature as a function of time for four sites in 2 dogs undergoing WBH. □, ○, dog 1; ●, △, dog 2 (Thrall et al. 1986)

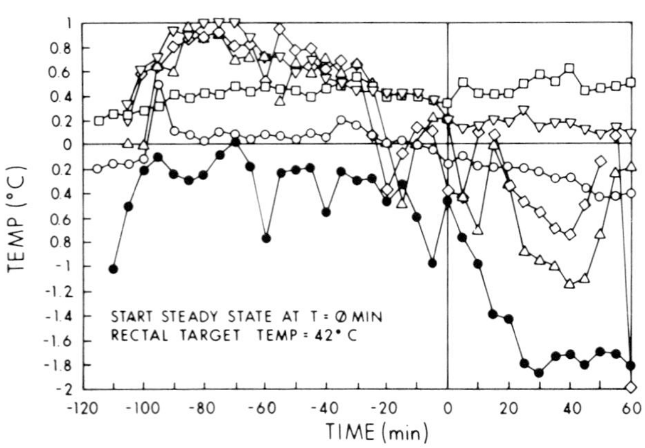

Fig. 12. Intratumoral temperature minus rectal temperature as a function of time at six sites in four dogs undergoing WBH. □, brachial tumor; △, right oral mucosal tumor; ○, brachial tumor; ●, oral tumor; ◇, left oral mucosal tumor; ▽, oral tumor (Thrall et al. 1986)

tery temperatures to rectal temperatures for a human undergoing systemic hyperthermia. Similarly, Fig. 8 illustrates the relationship of esophageal temperature to rectal temperature. Comparisons of Figs. 7, 8, and 9 illustrate the point that a properly placed insulated axillary temperature probe approximates blood temperature during the heating phase of WBH performed with an external heating device. Figures 10 and 11, as well as Fig. 5, provide the reader with data (derived

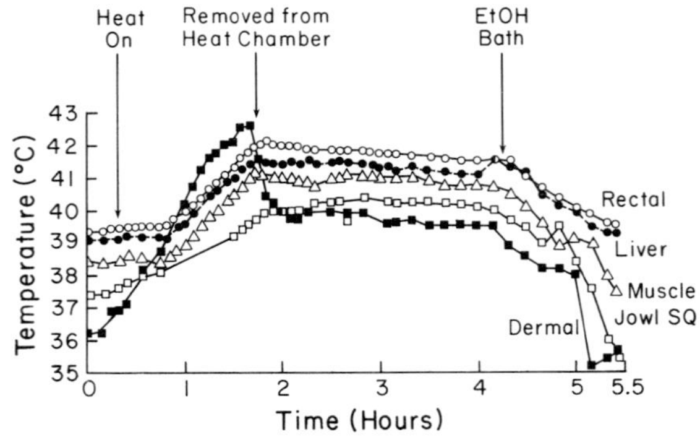

Fig. 13. Data obtained from a pig undergoing radiant heat systemic hyperthermia. *EtOH*, ethanol; *SQ*, Subcutaneous (Modified after Robins et al. 1983b)

from canine experiments) demonstrating the temperature relationship of various organ sites during WBH. Figure 12 demonstrates intratumoral temperatures obtained in a dog during WBH. The last figure in this series (Fig. 13) relates data obtained from a porcine animal model and demonstrates differences in deep visceral temperatures versus subcutaneous temperatures in an animal species which lacks sweat glands.

5.3 Cardiorespiratory Effects of WBH

The physiology of cardiovascular responses to externally applied heat (or exercise) in relation to thermoregulation have been detailed by Rowell (1983). One must be cautious, however, in directly extrapolating from the physiological responses described in unanesthetized healthy volunteers to responses found in a heterogeneous population of anesthetized, or heavily sedated cancer patients undergoing WBH in a variety of systems.

With the reservations described above, a brief outline of the normal cardiovascular thermoregulatory responses to externally applied heat follows. An elevation of environmental temperature is detected by "receptors" in the skin (free nerve endings) (Houdas and Ring 1982). A local axon reflex causes inhibition or the resting sympathetic vasoconstrictor tone of the smooth muscle cells of the glomera (subpapillary AV anastomoses). In addition, chemical mediators, e.g., kallikrein or bradykinin, may directly induce vasodilation, thereby contributing to the reduced peripheral vascular resistance. The net result is both increased cutaneous blood flow and cutaneous blood volume, the latter due to filling of the dense network of the subpapillary venous plexus. Neural impulses from peripheral cutaneous heat receptors travel to the hypothalamus and there reflexively cause: (a) sympathetic vasoconstriction of the splanchnic, muscle, and renal circulation, and (b) increased sympathetic output to the heart, thereby increasing heart rate and contractility. The increased heart rate, which occurs rapidly after the onset of heating, and the reduced peripheral vascular resistance combine to produce an increased cardiac output, while stroke volume is little changed (Houdas and Ring 1982). The skin receives most of the increased cardiac output and cutaneous blood flow may rise from 0.2 to 0.5 l/min to 7 l/min (Rowell 1983). The increased cardiac output does not completely compensate for the reduced peripheral vascular resistance and mean arterial blood pressure may fall slightly. Warmed blood returning to the heart heats the "core", and thus the central hypothalamic thermoreceptor, causing a further reflex boost to heart rate. Several investigators have shown that in the supine position, skin blood flow and heart rate correlate better with core temperature than with skin temperature (Rowell 1983), although the thermal reactivity of the vascular bed to the environment varies over different parts of the body (Houdas and Ring 1982). To compensate for the heat gained from the environment, reflexes via the hypothalamus and sympathetic nerves stimulate the sweat glands.

The majority of reported WBH clinical studies have involved some form of general anesthesia or marked sedation, in some cases requiring ventilatory support (Barlogie et al. 1979; Blair and Levin 1978; Larkin et al. 1977; Parks et al. 1979; Pettigrew and Ludgate 1977; Bull et al. 1979a; Ostrow et al. 1981). Somewhat different is the radiant heat system for WBH employed by Robins et al. (1985b) where only sedation is used. This methodology obviates the high skin temperatures at the onset of WBH which may cause cutaneous sympathetic stimulation as well as patient distress.

All groups have reported an increase in heart rate with increasing esophageal temperature (see Table 2). Pettigrew et al. (1974b) noted that while the maximum heart rate achieved was independent of the rate of core heating, faster heating (up to 6 °C/h) was attended by a lag or slower acceleration of heart rate. Mean heart rates at peak temperature are reported to range 131 beats/min (Barlogie et al. 1979) to 172 beats/min (Herman et al. 1982b). Although absolute figures vary, fairly good correlation is obtained when the changes are expressed as change in the pulse rate per 1 °C rise of body temperature. One survey of the literature estimated the mean change as 11.7 beats/min/°C (±0.73 SEM) (Van der Zee et al. 1987). Tachyarrhythmias have been seen by some workers (15% in Larkin's series, 1979); fewer occurred in the series of Barlogie et al. (1979) and Herman et al. (1982), and none were seen in the Bull series (Bull et al. 1979a) or in Robins' radiant heat phase I trial (Robins et al. 1985b). Ventricular arrhythmias were seen by Bull et al. (1979b) when WBH was combined with doxorubicin. Of interest, premature ventricular contractions (PVCs) reported by Larkin (1979) were difficult to control with lidocaine, and fatal ventricular fibrillation in patients treated by Euller-Rolle et al. (1978) prompted institution of the β-blocker, pindolol, once the pulse rose to 120 beats/min. (It should be noted that the use of β-blockers in the setting of WBH is po-

Table 2. Cardiovascular changes during WBH

	Pulse rate	Mean BP (*); pulse pressure (+)	Arrhythmias	CVP/PCWP	Cardiac output	O_2 consumption (+); alv-art O_2 gradient (*)
Pettigrew et al. (1974a)	↑	↔ +		↑	↑	
Larkin (1977, 1979)	↑	↑ +	+		↑	+ ↑
Euller-Rolle et al. (1978)	↑		+		↑	
Levin and Blair (1978)	↑	↑ +		↑	↑	
Barlogie et al. (1979)	↑	↑ +	+		↑	
Bull et al. (1979a)	↑		–		↑	
Kim et al. (1979b)	↑	↓ *		↓	↑	
Parks et al. (1979)	↑			↔	↑	* ↑
Ostrow et al. (1981)	↑	↑ +			↑	
Guntupali and Sladen (1982)	↑	↓ *		↑	↑	+ ↑
Herman et al. (1982c)	↑	↓ *	+		↑	* ↑
Faithful et al. (1984)	↑	↓ *			↑	
Robins et al. (1985a, b)	↑	↔ *	–	↔	↑	+ ↑
Van der Zee et al. (1987)	↑				↑	+ ↑

BP, blood pressure; CVP, central venous pressure; PCWP, pulmonary capillary wedge pressure; alv-art, alveolar-arterial; ↑, ↓, ↔, increase, decrease, or no change in parameter.

tentially dangerous. This is discussed in detail later in this section.) PVCs occurring in patients of Parks and Barlogie, however, responded promptly to lidocaine. Peak heart rate noted in the Wisconsin radiant heat system at 41.8 °C was ~150 beats/min and no arrhythmias occurred (Robins et al. 1985 b); all patients had an infusion of lidocaine running throughout the treatment.

Anesthetic drugs may reduce systolic blood pressure prior to the onset of hyperthermia (Pettigrew et al. 1974a; Kim et al. 1979b). During the WBH treatment itself, the reported systolic and mean arterial blood pressures varied widely. Levin and Blair (1978), using the Pettigrew wax technique, reported increased systolic and decreased diastolic pressures (e.g., widening of the pulse pressure), but Pettigrew himself noticed little change in the diastolic pressure (Pettigrew et al. 1974). Widening of the pulse pressure was also noticed by Ostrow et al. (1981) and Larkin's group (1977). Robins et al. (1985) reported no significant change in mean arterial pressure, unlike the reductions reported by others (Faithful et al. 1984; Herman et al. 1982c; Sladen et al. 1981; Guntupalli and Sladen 1982; Kim et al. 1979a). The experience with the radiant heat system (Robins et al. 1985) at Wisconsin also showed a widening of the pulse pressure when blood pressure cuffs were used for monitoring; however, this widening was significantly less marked when arterial lines were used. Barlogie's patients had a reduced diastolic but unchanged systolic blood pressure (Barlogie et al. 1979). Although peripheral vascular resistance and cardiac output were not measured in all series, the variety in blood pressure responses noted probably reflects differences in direct skin heating and vasodilatation, rate of heating, concentrations of anesthetic agents and sedative drugs, and rate and type of intravenous fluid replacement. These same factors may account for the reduced central venous pressure (CVP) noted by Kim et al. (1979a), while other workers reported a rise in CVP (Pettigrew et al. 1974; Sladen et al. 1981; Levin and Blair 1978). Those who have reported a reduced CVP similarly reported a lowered left ventricular filling pressure (pulmonary capillary wedge pressure, PCWP) (Kim et al. 1979b). Pulmonary artery pressures and PCWPs were relatively constant in the studies of Parks et al. (1979) and Robins et al. (1985).

Elevated cardiac output or cardiac index has been universally reported, rises generally being greater than 100%. Where reported, this elevation in cardiac output has correlated closely with heart rate, while stroke volume remained constant (Sladen et al. 1981; Robins et al. 1985) (see Fig. 14). Reductions in peripheral vascular resistance have been documented by Sladen et

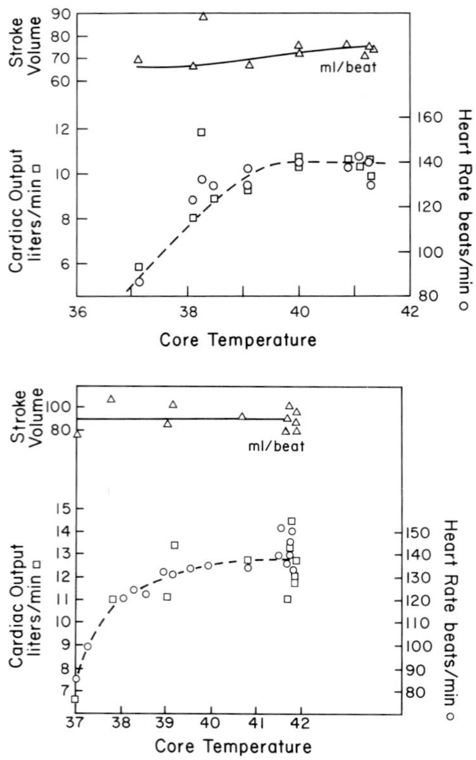

Fig. 14. Data from two different patients undergoing systemic hyperthermia with a radiant heat device. Cardiac output and heart rate are plotted as a function of rectal temperature. Heart rate becomes maximal between 39°–40°C. Cardiac output changes as a correlate of heart rate; hence, stroke volume remains relatively constant

al. (1981) and Faithfull et al. (1982). Faithfull's group has shown that the falling peripheral vascular resistance during heating, and hence lowered mean arterial pressure, accounted for the disparity between the elevated cardiac index and the reduced left ventricular work index (Faithfull et al. 1982). In addition, they reported elevated pulmonary arterial pressures and right ventricular work index, suggesting that in their system more strain was placed on the right than on the left ventricle during WBH.

There are few detailed reports on the cardiovascular status of patients following WBH. Van der Zee et al. (1987), using the POMP Siemens Cabinet, recorded a significantly elevated heart rate for 3 h after return to normal body temperature. Pulmonary artery pressure (raised during WBH) returned to baseline levels about 10 h after WBH, but mean systemic arterial pressure remained below baseline for at least 18 h after treatment (the final measurement timepoint).

Herman et al. (1982c) reported 30 WBH treatments – 16 using warming blankets and 14 using extracorporeal circulation – and in 7 instances noted mean blood pressure decreases to 60–70 mmHg for up to 2.5 h after treatment. They also noted that decreases of mean blood pressure, occurring at elevated temperatures, were accentuated at the end of therapy when patients were actively cooled. Herman infused the α-agonist phenylephrine during the cooling period to prevent hypotension.

Pettigrew et al. (1974a) observed that a persistent tachycardia with low blood pressure could develop in patients with "sensitive" tumors. Barlogie et al. (1979) commenting on the diastolic pressure (which had decreased during treatment), noted a rapid return to normal during the ensuing 12 h, while Bull et al. (1979a) noted that 5 out of 14 patients had systolic blood pressures between 70 and 90 mmHg and 90 mmHg for 30 min–3 h after treatment.

When reported, oxygen consumption rose consistently during WBH (Robins et al. 1985b; Sladen et al. 1981; Van der Zee et al. 1987). Robins et al. (1985b) noted that as core temperature increased, a rise in oxygen consumption occurred consistent with an increase in metabolic rate. Arterial and venous oxygen saturation remained normal, even in patients not receiving nasal oxygen. Arterial O_2 tension also remained normal during treatment.

In the studies reported by Van der Zee et al. 1987, both oxygen flux (calculated as cardiac output × arterial oxygen content) and oxygen consumption (cardiac output × arteriomixed venous oxygen content difference) were measured. Both parameters appeared little affected by anesthesia induction, but were significantly increased during heating and at plateau temperature. These workers emphasized particularly an examination of the ratio of these two parameters rather than concentrating merely on the absolute values for either. They showed that during the early warming phase of WBH, oxygen extraction or utilization was relatively smaller than oxygen flux, suggesting that oxygen needs are more than fully met during hyperthermia treatment. However, analysis of alveolar-arterial oxygen gradients is complicated by the variations in anesthetic technique. Larkin et al. (1977), Herman et al. (1982c), and Parks et al. (1979) all reported elevated gradients, which suggest some intrapulmonary shunting and/or pulmonary edema. Improvements were noted by Herman and Parks when positive end expiratory pressure (PEEP) was given. Bull's patients, breathing spontaneously during WBH, experienced mild hyperventilation and respiratory alkalosis (Bull et al. 1979a).

Reports of Lees et al. (1982) and Kim et al. (1979b) have confirmed in cancer patients the physiological concepts of cardiovascular adaptation to heat stress defined by Rowell (1983). They demonstrated that the redistribution of blood flow away from the splanchnic to the cutaneous circulation correlated with lower levels of cutaneous venous norepinephrine during WBH, at a time when mixed venous levels were elevated.

Circulatory and respiratory stresses in cancer patients undergoing WBH are significant. As heart rates in excess of 150 beats/min are often observed during WBH, the existence of a preexisting coronary disease remains a contraindication to WBH treatment (Robins and Neville 1986). As mentioned above, Euler-Rolle et al. (1978) suggested that β-blockers might be cardioprotective. Parks (pers. comm., 1986) found that use of β-blockers with extracorporeal WBH precipitated cardiac decompensation. In this regard, two studies, each utilizing a canine model, have suggested that β-blockers might, in fact, be deleterious during WBH. Milnor et al. (1966) (reported in Van der Zee et al. 1987) demonstrated that pulmonary blood flow could be increased with less input power if the pulse rate increased while the stroke volume remained constant. Thus, it can be concluded that high pulse rates might prevent excessive rises in right ventricular work in patients undergoing WBH, and artificially reducing the heart rate would be inappropriate.

Robins et al. (1991a) treated dogs with WBH in a radiant heat system analogous to the clinical WBH they described (Robins et al. 1985b). When the animals were at 42 °C plateau temperature, propranolol was administered intravenously. In one example, an animal showed a fall in cardiac ejection fraction from 52% to 45% associated with a 13% decrease in heart rate, within 5 min of total propranolol administration. At this time, nuclear scanning demonstrated changes in pulmonary vasculature and lung volume indicative of early pulmonary edema. By cooling the animal to 39 °C, these changes reversed and ejection fraction improved to 54%. These studies also demonstrated reductions in mean blood pressure, cardiac output, and stroke volume after using β-blockades during WBH in dogs. These results argue for a relative contraindication to drug-induced β-blockade during WBH, and certainly if β-blockers are administered, invasive hemodynamic monitoring appears mandatory.

Since the completion of these dog studies, patients presenting for WBH at the University of Wisconsin Clinical Cancer Center who are already receiving β-blockers for hypertension are first evaluated with an exercise, nuclear ventriculogram. The patients are then switched from β-blockers to captopril with or without diuretics. They are then restudied by nuclear ventriculography at least 1 month later. Only those patients demonstrating physiologic increases in heart rate, blood pressure, and ejection fraction are eligible for study. In patients with longstanding essential hypertension, thallium scanning appears useful as an additional screening test for coronary artery disease (Robins et al. 1989a).

WBH thus exerts a significant effect on all parameters of the cardiovascular system. The net cardiovascular changes observed during clinical WBH are, however, as much the result of the methodology of hyperthermia induction as the effects of thermal stress itself, which explains the variation in the cardiovascular responses observed.

5.4 Biochemical Effects of WBH

A fairly consistent pattern (with exceptions to be noted) of biochemical and electrolyte changes occurs during and after 41 °–42 °C systemic hyperthermia. In patients receiving dextrose in intravenous solutions hyperglycemia is always observed. This is in part related to the volume and rate of intravenous dextrose given. A secondary consideration is the release of adrenocorticotropic hormone (ACTH) and cortisol (Parks et al. 1978; Robins et al. 1987a, b) as well as catecholamines (Kim et al. 1979a) which occurs with WBH. Additionally, others (Burmeister et al. 1980) have shown rises in glycogen and a decrease in insulin. In assessing the effect of WBH on serum potassium (K^+) it is essentially impossible to distinguish changes related to urinary excretion, acid-base balance, sweating, and the rate of intravenous replacement. Both Pettigrew et al. (1974) and Larkin et al. (1977) noted rises in serum K^+ followed by falls at 24 h. Other workers reported decreases in K^+ during WBH requiring replacement (Barlogie et al. 1979; Van der Zee et al. 1982; Parks et al. 1979; Ostro et al. 1981; Robins et al. 1985). Parks et al. (1979) reported increased losses of magnesium (Mg), calcium (Ca), and phosphate (PO_4). These observations were consistent with the fall of serum ions observed both by Parks and most other investigators (Larkin et al. 1977; Bull et al. 1979; Barlogie et al. 1979; Ostrow et al. 1981; Herman et al. 1982). Other workers (in contrast to Parks), however, using WBH systems other than the extracorporeal approach used by Parks, have not found elevated urinary or stool losses of Ca, PO_4, or Mg. Factors which may relate to these differing experiences may include the use of furosemide during extracorporeal WBH, or electrolyte shifts caused by changing pH (alkalotic) associated with WBH systems encompassing general anesthesia and mechanical ventilation. Beyond this, ion shifts have been observed in patients maintained at a pH of 7.4; thus, another as yet unidentified effect of WBH may be a contributing factor. Of note, patients treated with radiant heat WBH often develop a mild respiratory acidosis, which reflects their respiratory rate and/or degree of sedation; these patients however have not been observed to acquire clinically significant changes in sodium (Na^+), K^+, Ca, Mg, or PO_4 (Robins and Neville 1986).

Clearly the acid-base changes which occur during WBH reflect both the respiratory status of the patient as well as increased metabolic work. Mechanical ventilation during WBH typically results in alkalosis, although some (Sladen et al. 1981) have observed increases in lactic acid and acidosis. Interestingly, Robins et al. (1988a) did not observe such changes using radiant heat WBH even in combination with lonidamine, a chemotherapeutic drug which predisposes to increases in systemic lactic acid levels. Faithfull et al. (1982) reported no significant pH changes during WBH; these workers found the same decreases in Mg, PO_4, and Ca discussed above; they noted, however, that decreases in Ca were related to a fall in serum protein, while ionized calcium remained normal. Neumann et al. (1988) have accrued limited data to suggest an increase in plasma acetate levels in patients undergoing 40 °C WBH using the Sieman box (see Table 1). The monitoring of venous plasma acetate has not been attempted by other groups. Neumann et al. (1988) speculated that the release of acetate was from neoplastic tissue. This situation may be comparable to that of lactic dehydrogenase (LDH) which is discussed below.

Generally speaking, most groups have not reported detailed information relating to renal function. Lees et al. (1982) presented data consistent with diminished renal blood flow during WBH. There is a general consensus that at 42 °C hourly urine output significantly falls. Bull et al. (1979) did not find changes in creatinine clearance or serum creatinine 24 h after WBH. Robins et al. (1985) observed minor elevations of serum creatinine after 41.8 °C WBH, but no changes in creatinine clearance values (Robins and Neville 1986). These observations are consistent with an increased release of creatinine during radiant heat WBH. Clearly, renal compromise is possible during WBH. For example, Faithfull et al. (1982) have observed significant falls in urine output with associated increase in urea and blood urea nitrogen. Such observations suggest that it is wise to avoid potentially renal toxic agents, e.g., aminoglycosides, during systemic hyperthermia. Skeletal muscle-derived creatinine phosphokinase (CPK) has been shown to rise sporadically in various systems for WBH (Robins et al. 1985; Parks et al. 1979; Barlogie et al. 1979). For radiant heat WBH, CPK rises have been noted in less than 1% of treat-

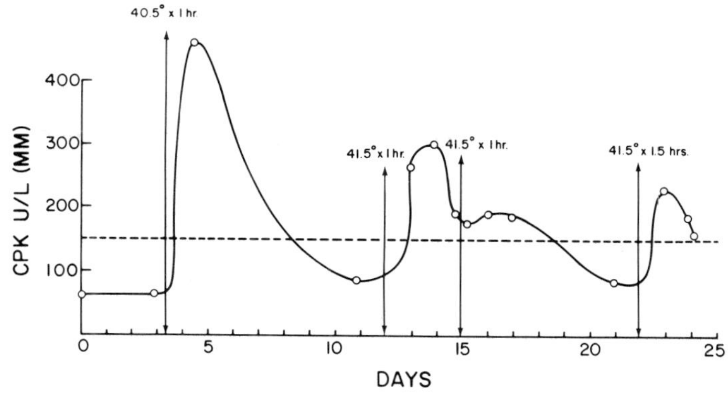

Fig. 15. Release of skeletal muscle enzyme in a patient undergoing three successive systemic hyperthermia treatments. An apparent thermal adaptation occurred in this patient with regard to creatinine phosphokinase (*CPK*) release

ments. We have noted that when this does occur, subsequent treatments – even at higher temperatures or longer durations – are associated with quantitatively smaller rises in serum CPK. This is graphically illustrated in Fig. 15. Muscle damage encountered during WBH with some WBH methodologies may relate in part to significantly reduced serum PO_4 levels; marked hypophosphatemia has been associated with rhadomyolysis as well as neurological deficits (Knochel 1977). The changes in phosphorus levels during WBH are clearly method dependent. Guntupalli et al. (1984), utilizing a technique in which patients are immersed in hot water, concluded that the hypophosphatemia they observed was related to a decreased tubular reabsorptive capacity. Their observation was consistent with a decrease in the renal threshold for phosphorus reabsorption to low levels during WBH – with a return to baseline after WBH. This result is not consistent with the experience gained with other methodologies (Parks et al. 1979; Bull et al. 1979; Robins et al. 1985). Parks et al. (1979) observed increased urinary phosphorus excretion for up to 96 h after WBH. Bull et al. (1979), on the other hand, reported no increase in phosphorus excretion. Differences in clinical results may relate to hyperventilation and associated respiratory alkalosis associated with some WBH systems, e.g., Bull et al. (1979). It is of interest to note that the changes reported for phosphorus excretion noted by Guntupalli et al. (1984) were independent of changes in urinary cyclic AMP excretion, arterial CO_2 tension, or circulating parathyroid hormone level. (A full discussion of the hormonal changes of WBH follows below.)

Abnormalities of liver function tests (LFT), i.e., serum hepatic enzyme levels, have been reported for many of the WBH systems. Of the enzymes measured, LDH rose most consistently. Bull et al. (1979) and Barlogie et al. (1979), however, reported no change in this enzyme. Robins et al. (1985) pointed out the need to fractionate this enzyme, particularly if a rise in LDH is observed in the absence of other LFT abnormalities. This group found that the liver-associated LDH fraction, i.e., 5, was rarely increased; rises in LDH were invariably associated with hyperthermia-induced tumor lysis syndromes. Thus, elevations were observed in the neoplastic associated fractions 3 and 4. Robins' group has found that metastatic disease involving the liver is highly predisposed to hyperthermic killing; this is discussed more fully elsewhere (Robins 1991a). Because patients may evolve passive congestion due to tumor lysis, and because of the overall sensitivity of the liver to thermal injury, the Wisconsin group as a rule restricts patient entry to patients in whom hepatic replacement by tumor is less than one-third, and LFT are less than twice normal. Most groups have reported transaminase rises (Pettigrew et al. 1974; Larkin et al. 1977; Levin and Blair 1978; Blair and Levin 1978; Ostrow et al. 1981; Herman et al. 1982). Levin and Blair (1978) as well as Larkin et al. (1977) noted that changes were less pronounced with subsequent WBH treatment; they suggest some form of thermal adaptation had occurred. This might be similar to the situation for CPK discussed above. Transient elevations of bilirubin have also been noted (Parks et al. 1979; Sladen et al. 1981; Levin and Blair 1978; Pettigrew et al. 1974b). It would appear that alkaline phosphatase abnormalities may take longer to resolve than transaminase changes (Larkin et al. 1977). Our review of the literature suggests that changes in bilirubin may be the most ominous prognosticator of hepatic damage. Cases of significant hepatic necrosis have been seen by several groups (Pettigrew et al. 1974b; Levin and Blair 1978; Van der Zee et al. 1982; Herman et al. 1982). Our group has not encountered hepatic damage in over 700 treatments. This may relate to the hepatic restrictions discussed above, as well as the avoidance of heat-drug interactions which occur with full general anesthesia (avoided by the University of Wisconsin's approach to WBH [Robins et al. 1985]). In this regard, it should be noted that Herman et al. (1982) did observe tumor necrosis in the absence of hepatic tumor involvement.

Finally, it appears that the chronic use of hepatotoxins, e.g., alcohol or phenobarbital, may predispose patients to thermal hepatic damage (Pettigrew et al. 1974b; Levin and Blair 1984). (Our group restricts alcohol ingestion in all patients receiving WBH.)
Much of the above discussion (regarding both normal hepatocytes as neoplastic involvement of the liver, being extremely sensitive to hyperthermia effects) is consistent with a special metabolic milieu in the liver which mitigates against the development of thermal tolerance. Consistent with this hypothetical view is a study by Prionos et al. (1985) in a canine model.

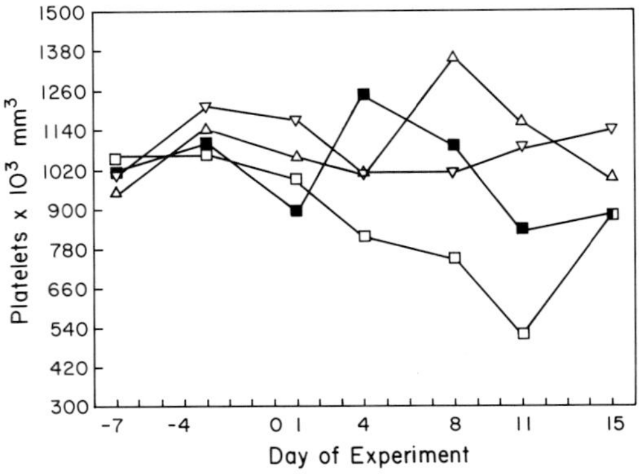

Fig. 16. The protective effect of WBH (△) and TBI-induced thrombocytopenia (□) in a mouse model. Untreated control (CON; ▽) values are also shown. A similar phenomena was observed in a patient receiving TBI-WBH treatment (■) for nodular B cell neoplasms (Modified after Robins et al. 1990a)

5.5 Hematological Changes

The effect of WBH on leukocyte function has previously been reviewed in Chap. 2. Neutropenia in association with WBH is invariably related to adjunctive radiotherapy and/or chemotherapy. Neutrophilia, on the other hand, is undoubtedly related in part to rises in ACTH and cortisol and catecholamine. The relationship of WBH to platelet count has recently been found to be complex and worthy of further investigation. Several systems for WBH have been associated with falls in platelet counts, without evidence of associated disseminated intravascular coagulation (DIC) (Larkin et al. 1977; Levin and Blair 1978; Barlogie et al. 1979; Parks et al. 1979; Van der Zee et al. 1982; Herman et al. 1982a). The possible relationship to chemotherapy in some of these reports is not clear. Parks et al. (1979) reported drops in platelet counts over prolonged time durations. Interestingly, however, both Bull et al. (1979) and Robins et al. (1985) found no evidence of thrombocytopenia when using systems involving sedation (in contrast to general anesthesia and mechanical ventilation). Further, Bull et al. (1979) and Robins et al. (1985) found no evidence of coagulopathies in contrast to others whose patients did show evidence of DIC (Levin and Blair 1978; Barlogie et al. 1979; Van der Zee 1982; Herman et al. 1982a; Sladen et al. 1981).
Recently, Robins et al. (1990a) have reported the apparent protective properties of 41.8 °C radiant heat WBH in relationship to radiation-induced thrombocytopenia in this clinical setting. Their experiments using a murine model reinforced this presumptive clinical observation (see Fig. 16). If additional clinical work confirms this finding, the most obvious explanation relates to the release of a WBH-induced hematopoietic factor. Relative to this a recent murine study has shown the 40 °C WBH induction of interleukin-1 (Shen et al. 1991; see also Dinarello et al. 1985).

Hemoglobin values have dropped in some WBH series and are not reported in others. This phenomenon appears to be related in most cases to hemodilution associated with intravenous fluids, and in some cases, frequent phlebotomy related to medical and investigative testing. Hemolysis has not been reported as a significant complication of systemic hyperthermia. In this regard, Whang-Peng et al. (1981) have studied erythrocyte fragility in patients undergoing WBH with and without chemotherapy and have found no significant abnormalities.

5.6 Neurological Sequelae

Most patients undergoing systemic hyperthermia have had previous exposure to chemotherapy and/or ionizing irradiation. Radiation and chemotherapeutic drugs such as platinum agents, and vinca alkaloids, have a clear potential for neurologic sequelae. In this context peripheral neuropathies have been associated with WBH. Most of the patients of Barlogie, Bull, Herman, and Larkin (see Table 1) who developed peripheral neuropathy had previously received antineoplastic agents. Thus, it is possible that the WBH might have exacerbated or precipitated a previously subclinical neuropathy. (In this regard our group excludes patients with preexisting peripheral neuropathies from WBH treatment.)
A polyneuropathy resembling Guillain-Barré syndrome was reported in three patients receiving WBH in conjunction with the nitrosourea BCNU (Selker et al. 1983). Among the most serious neurological toxici-

ties observed following WBH was acute transverse myelitis in three patients reported by Parks' group (Douglas et al. 1981). All three patients had received radiation to the spinal cord and had a previous exposure to BCNU. The early time course in relationship to irradiation for the development of transverse myelitis (which developed shortly after WBH) clearly implicated WBH as a contributing factor in this catastrophic complication. However it is not possible to delineate the relative roles of temperature elevation per se, compared to hemodynamic or other changes related to WBH. In this regard, Neville et al. (1984) tried to sort out the possible contributing variables, i.e., WBH, radiation, and BCNU using a rat model. Unfortunately this model was not useful for replicating the precise clinical phenomena. (The reader is referred to this manuscript for a fuller treatment of this important issue. Many, but not all, researchers will exclude patients from WBH who have a previous history of spinal cord irradiation. It is relevant to this discussion that Robins et al. (1985) have reported a "radiation recall" phenomenon in a patient who received prior lymph node irradiation.)

Van der Zee et al. (1982) reported transient agitation and hyperexcitability after WBH in 19 patients; this observation was attributed to low magnesium levels discussed above. Clearly it is possible that transient muscle weakness observed after WBH may relate to reduced serum calcium, magnesium, or phosphate (Knochel 1977).

Dubois et al. (1980) at the National Cancer Institute conducted electroencephalograph (EEG) studies in a series of 21 patients undergoing WBH. They found a diffuse decrease in cortical activity at a core temperature of 41 °C, as reflected by tracing changes in amplitude and rhythmicity. EEG changes consistent with toxic or metabolic encephalopathy were noted above 41.5 °C. These workers reported no EEG evidence of seizure activity.

Seizure activity in WBH patients has been reported by Barlogie et al. (1979) and Herman et al. (1982). Most groups exclude patients with previous histories of seizure or intracranial lesions. (If intracranial disease is being addressed in the context of a protocol, then intracranial pressure monitoring is virtually mandatory. Parenthetically, in normal dogs undergoing WBH epidural pressure does not increase [Van Rhoon and Van der Zee 1983].) In addition, the patients receiving WBH with the radiant heat technology used by Robins et al. (1985) always receive a thiopental infusion. These workers believe such an infusion provides seizure prophylaxis. They have not observed any seizure problems in their series to date of more than 700 treatments.

5.7 Endocrine Function and WBH

Several groups have reported increases in plasma ACTH and cortisol after WBH (Parks et al. 1978; Burmeister et al. 1980; Beckley et al. 1982; Bull et al. 1982; Robins et al. 1987a). In a series of endocrine evaluations by Burmeister et al. (1980), increases in growth hormone, prolactin, glucagon, aldosterone, and plasma renin activity were reported. A minor decline in insulin was observed; no changes in follicle-stimulating hormone in (FSH), luteinizing hormone (LH), thyroid-stimulating hormone (TSH), gastrin, and thyroid hormones were noted. Kim et al. (1979a) and Cornau et al. (1984) found increases in catecholamine levels.

Robins et al. (1987a, b) noted pain relief after WBH treatment in a series of patients having no objective signs of tumor regression. (Indeed, many investigators

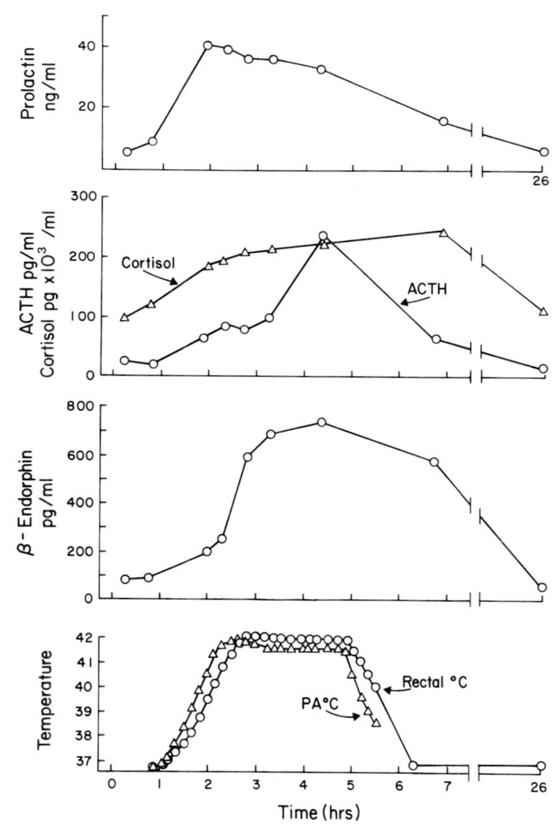

Fig. 17. Data were obtained from a 47-year-old white male with colon carcinoma metastatic to the liver. Rectal and pulmonary artery (*PA*) temperatures during WBH are shown in the *lower graph*. Included are time profiles for changes in plasma β-endorphin, adrenocorticotropic hormone (*ACTH*) and cortisol and prolactin. Zero time corresponds to 8:00 a.m. The patient's white blood cell count (cells/mm$^3 \times 10^{-3}$) was 6.5, 1 day prior to WBH; 6.0 peak temperature; 9.3, 1 day after WBH; and 11.3, 2 days after WBH (Robins et al. 1987a)

had noted pain relief after WBH and assumed this was putative evidence for a response.)

In this regard, as Guillemin et al. (1977) had noted, increases in ACTH occur in concert with rises in plasma β-endorphin levels. Therefore, Robins group elected to prospectively evaluate whether β-endorphin release was responsible for the pain relief observed in WBH patients not obtaining a clinical remission. These patients did exhibit thermal-induced increases in plasma levels of β-endorphin as well as prolactin, ACTH and cortisol. Figure 17 illustrates the time relationship of this hormonal release juxtaposed to a WBH treatment. Heat-induced release of pituitary hormones have also been reported for other species (Seigel et al. 1979; Schams et al. 1980). The relationship between thermal dose and the release of hormones is addressed in a report by Robins et al. (1987a).

5.8 Gastrointestinal Toxicity

As we have previously reviewed (Robins and Neville 1986), nausea, vomiting, and diarrhea are commonly reported side effects for some WBH methodologies. Diarrhea can be protracted, lasting up to 48 h in some instances (Ostrow 1981; Herman et al. 1982a).

Diarrhea or constipation has not been a complication in our experience with radiant heat WBH. About 20%–30% of patients will experience one or two episodes of vomiting 2–3 h after radiant heat WBH. This emesis, which is not associated with nausea, is probably related to gastric stasis caused by thiopental (see Sect. 5.6). In patients exhibiting this problem, metoclopramide is given prophylactically with excellent results (after WBH when the patients return to 37 °C).

Nonintubated patients receiving radiant heat WBH and emetogenic chemotherapy or radiation are at risk for aspiration pneumonia. In this clinical situation, we routinely add droperidol (1.25–4 mg) to our pharmacological approach to sedation, which also serves as a completely effective antiemetic. We have not had a single episode of vomiting during a WBH-chemotherapy treatment with this approach (Robins et al. 1991b).

5.9 Miscellaneous Toxicities

Careful positioning and support during WBH is critical to avoid skin burns and decubitus ulceration in systems requiring anesthetized patients. In this regard a clinitron bed is now standardly used at the University of Texas by Bull and her coworkers (Cornau et al. 1984). Pressure sores can easily develop in hyperthermic temperature. By way of example our group now routinely uses only an *ear* oximeter monitoring device as opposed to a *finger* oximeter (to measure O_2 saturation continuously during WBH); we observed mild superficial skin necrosis on a patient's fingertip after WBH due to the pressure of a finger oximeter. This would never occur under normothermic conditions.

The development of circumoral herpes simplex following WBH has been commonly reported following WBH (Pettigrew et al. 1974; Larkin et al. 1977; Bull et al. 1979; Barlogie et al. 1979). It has been our experience, and we assume the experience of others that this only occurs in patients with a previous history of cold sores. We have routinely placed patients with post-WBH herpes simplex lesions on acyclovir which has resulted in prompt resolution of the infection. We are not aware of reports of WBH precipitating herpes zoster.

A vague malaise and lethargy after WBH is observed almost universally. However, as discussed above, these symptoms can be simultaneously accompanied by a sence of well-being or pain relief due to endorphin release.

Posthyperthermia fever without infection has also been commonly described. Bull et al. (1979) have observed fevers up to 41 °C. In our experience this may be associated with evidence of tumor regression. Our group has commonly observed the triad of fever, increase in the tumor-related LDH fraction (3 and 4) (see Sect. 5.4), and hiccups in patients obtaining regression of liver metastasis.

Many authors in reviews have extrapolated from the physiological changes seen during heat stroke in discussing the toxicities or potential morbidity of WBH. We believe that such analogies are not valid and can result in erroneous conclusions. Heat stroke is a pathological state in which critical physiological variables, e.g., fluid status, are not controlled or maintained.

6 WBH Animal Studies

6.1 Introduction

Throughout this text we have presented the results of preclinical studies which were relevant to the topics being presented. In this chapter we wish to summarize some of the literature regarding in vivo WBH studies to serve as a convenient reference point for the reader to pursue further inquiry into the literature, or as a starting point for laboratory research.

Any animal model can be useful, as long as the investigator recognizes its limitations in the context of the question being addressed. By way of example, the thermal regulatory mechanisms of rodents are entirely different from those in large mammals (Robins et al. 1984c). Anesthetic agents cause a profound lowering of core temperature of rodents at normothermic temperatures. In this same regard, these species apparently do not increase their metabolic rates during systemic hyperthermia; hence they immediately cool after being removed from an environment designed to induce WBH. This is true in the absence and presence of anesthetic agents (Robins et al. 1984c).

This being the case, one might predict that murine systems are inappropriate to model WBH pharmacology. Indeed, although the results obtained with a canine model (Page et al. 1989) predicted the pharmacokinetics of carboplatin for humans (Robins et al. 1990b) during WBH, results obtained using rats were entirely different (Ono et al. 1990).

The above discussion is in no way meant to discourage the use of murine models in the setting of WBH. Actually, we have found that murine systems (Steeves et al. 1987; Robins et al. 1990a) are often closely predictive of clinical results (Robins et al. 1990a). Further, the availability of transplantable tumor models makes the use of rodents essential to ongoing preclinical WBH research.

In approaching the design of rodent research, we believe it is optimal to maximize results by evaluating both normal tissue and neoplastic cell toxicity whenever possible. This allows the investigator to estimate the effect of WBH on the therapeutic index and/or therapeutic gain. Examples of this approach appear in the literature (e.g., Honess and Bleehn 1985a; Steeves et al. 1987).

6.2 Large Animals

Both the pig (Dickson et al. 1979; Robins et al. 1983b) and the dog (Maxwell et al. 1959; Hugander et al. 1987; Thrall et al. 1989a, b; Macy et al. 1985; Robins 1988) have proven to provide excellent physiological models for systemic hyperthermia. Although the pig may represent the ideal physiological model, the ease of working with dogs, as well as the availability of spontaneous pet tumors make this species preferable for most routine studies. Parenthetically, there is a strain of miniature pig that develops a genetically destined spontaneous lymphoma syndrome (McTaggart et al. 1979; Brownlie et al. 1978) which might prove useful in WBH studies.

Other species on which systemic hyperthermia has been performed include monkeys, rabbits, and cats. The rabbit for which neoplastic models exist (Dickson and Shah 1977; Wile et al. 1983b) is an atypical model for WBH as the normal body temperature of this species is significantly above 37 °C (Robins 1988). Honda et al. (1988) reported results in Japanese monkeys. (The results in this study suggesting core temperatures of 43 °C may be quantitatively questionable, as there is no evidence that the authors calibrated their thermometry system.) Macy and Gasper (1988) have demonstrated the feasibility of performing WBH in cats, which may have significance in studying the effect of hyperthermia on retrovirus infections in a feline model (see also Sect. 3.1).

6.3 Murine Models

It appears that the physiological tolerance for WBH can vary with age, strain of animal, and the number of WBH treatments. In general, older animals, regardless of species (with the possible exception of properly screened humans), will encounter a greater degree of morbidity and mortality. It should be noted that different strains of mice will tolerate WBH quite differently. It is recommended, therefore, that the choice of a transplantable murine model for WBH be based in part on a preevaluation of a particular strain of mouse's physiological tolerance of systemic hyperthermia. It should be noted that rodents (and probably large mammals) tolerate WBH better after each successive WBH treatment. In this regard, the increased survival of mice and rats after an initial WBH treatment relative to successive treatments – termed thermal tolerance by some (Li and Hahn 1983; Kapp and Lord 1983) – we regard as a gross physiological adaptation, and not necessarily "thermal tolerance" at the cellular level (Steeves et al. 1982; Hahn 1982; Henle and Dethlefsen 1978).

We have previously reviewed various techniques for inducing WBH in rodents (Robins and Neville 1986). Techniques range from a hot air blower (Yerushalmi 1976) and hot air (Wright 1976) to hot water (Hofer et al. 1976; Wondergem et al. 1988). Radiant heat *without* anesthesia (Robins 1984) is now used by several groups.

6.4 Special Considerations

6.4.1 Species Differences

As previously discussed, the dog has been and will undoubtedly continue to be a valuable model for WBH. Pet tumors offer a special opportunity to conduct phase II and phase III trials (Dewhirst et al. 1982; Dewhirst and Sim 1984b). This species, however, can present unusual problems relative to the metabolism of drugs. For example, lonidamine, which can be given to humans orally in the context of WBH (Robins et al. 1988a), has a peculiar metabolism in the gastrointestinal tract of dogs and must be given intravenously (Price et al. 1989). The metabolism of Adriamycin has been shown to be different in dogs (Wilke et al. 1991) and rabbits (Mimnaugh et al. 1978). In this same regard, the use of body surface area in the dog to determine drug delivery can also be problematic (Page et al. 1988). The effect of various anesthetic agents has been studied in detail in dogs (Hugander et al. 1987; Meyer et al. 1986) and must be taken into consideration. Beyond this, the use of insulation to reduce extremity temperature nonuniformity is also a factor in working with this species, which may be relevant to other species – including humans (Thrall et al. 1987, 1989a).

6.4.2 WBH and Metastatic Dissemination

In the context of this chapter on in vivo models, it is relevant to point out that the issue of hyperthermia stimulating metastatic spread has been raised in three species. Yerushalmi (1976) and Shah and Dickson (1978b) demonstrated increased metastasis utilizing immunogenic models in the mouse and rabbit respectively. This observation has *not* been confirmed with other models (Marmor et al. 1977; Kim and Hahn 1979; Steeves et al. 1987). In a murine study by Wile et al. (1983b) survival was used as an end point in evaluating WBH alone and WBH and cisplatin. The decreased survival seen in the combination arm may have been due to renal toxicity, rather than the untested assumption on the part of the authors of increased tumor progression. Certainly, as is discussed in Chap. 4, cisplatin nephrotoxicity is markedly enhanced by WBH.

A report by Lord et al. (1981) focused on the treatment of spontaneous osteosarcoma in pet dogs. Clearly this should be an appropriate model to address the issue of increased metastasis. In this nonrandomized series, animals receiving WBH had increased metastatic disease involving bone, rather than lung which is a more typical site. Thus, a reasonable interpretation of this report might be that the survival of the dogs was increased leading to an alteration of the natural history of the disease. Such an analogous clinical scenario would be the increased incidence of CNS disease (a sanctuary site for chemotherapy) in patients being treated successfully with antineoplastic drugs. A report by Neville et al. (1986) involving the WBH treatment of a patient with pancreatic cancer provides another possible example of this phenomenon, i.e., control of local disease resulting in a new anatomic pattern of metastatic spread. The only other information which may be relevant to this report by Lord et al. (1981) relates to bone marrow temperature in the dog during WBH. The bone marrow temperature of the dog can be up to several tenths of a degree lower than core temperature during the plateau phase of WBH (Thrall et al. 1986; Hugander et al. 1987).

In summary, from a preclinical standpoint, the relationship of WBH to metastatic spread would be best defined by a randomized study involving WBH as a single modality involving a spontaneous nonimmunogenic model. Again, the reader is reminded that the ultimate utilization of WBH in humans and animals (i.e., pets) resides in its use as an adjunct to other forms of therapy. In the limited experience with WBH as an adjunct to radiation (Robins et al. 1990a) and chemotherapy (Englehardt 1984) in which there is an appropriate control group, there is no indication that WBH shortens survival or increases metastasis; rather just the opposite is the case.

7 Special Consideration for the Future

7.1 Nononcological Considerations

7.1.1 Collagen Vascular Diseases

With the availability of nontoxic systems for WBH in carefully selected patients (Robins 1984; Robins et al. 1989a), the potential for utilizing systemic hyperthermia in nononcological settings presents itself. The collagen vascular diseases represent an area of special interest in this regard. We have anecdotally observed significant improvements in various incidental arthritic conditions in cancer patients undergoing WBH. Although this may be in part a reflection of WBH-induced β-endorphin release (Robins et al. 1987a, b), these observations could be explored in the context of phase I and phase II studies.

Consistent with this concept, Noodleman et al. (1984) have reported the use of local hyperthermia in treating psoriatic plaques. The skin temperatures achieved during the heating phase of radiant heat WBH (and probably other transcutaneous methodologies) are adequate to treat patients with severe psoriasis. As this disease has systemic manifestations, such a clinical trial might prove relevant in regard to other therapeutic effects, e.g., relative to psoriatic arthritis.

7.1.2 Hypothermia

The rescue of exposure victims with accidental hypothermia continues to represent a significant medical problem. Hypothermia is defined as the unintentional lowering of body core temperature below 35 °C (Golden 1972; Pozos and Wittmers 1983); in (a) mild cases – 33 °–35 °C – the patient is conscious but confused and shivering is usually present; in (b) moderate cases – 30 °–33 °C – the patient is often unconscious or very drowsy and shivering is present; and in (c) severe cases – <30 °C – the patient is usually unconscious and at high risk for cardiac arrhythmias with shivering ceased or markedly diminished.

In general, the mortality rates in treating hypothermic victims in large series have approached 50% (Pozos and Wittmers 1983; Bowman 1977; Gregory and Doolittle 1973). Bowman has estimated the risk of fatality for mild hypothermia to be 25%; for moderate cases, 32%, and severe cases, 66%. In spite of various rewarming strategies, mildly hypothermic patients with core temperatures in the range of 33.9 °–35 °C have mortality rates as high as 30% (Pozos and Wittmers 1983). Although many approaches to rewarming therapy have been used, there is still a general consensus that a more effective technique is required (Pozos and Wittmers 1983). Comparison of various methodologies indicates no statistical advantage to any given system. It has been claimed that the success of all systems is poor. Techniques which have been utilized to date include: (a) hot water immersion, (b) heated inhaled air, (c) hot water blanket, (d) peritoneal dialysis, (e) diathermy, (f) thoracic or gastric lavage, and (g) extracorporeal heating (Pozos and Wittmers 1983; Reuler 1978; Webb 1973; Collis et al. 1977; Hayward and Steinman 1975; Fernandez et al. 1970; Bigelow et al. 1952; Blair et al. 1977; Pickering et al. 1977; Wickstrom et al. 1976; Patton and Doolittle 1972; Gregory et al. 1973).

In reviewing this problem in the light of knowledge gained from hyperthermia experience, we project an ideal rewarming technology should include:

1. Accurate thermometry in the hypothermic range
2. The potential to initiate therapy immediately. (Invasive techniques, e.g., extracorporeal heating, require time during which the patient can become progressively more hypothermic secondary to a falling basal metabolic rate.)
3. The potential to monitor patients, e.g., blood pressure, ECG rhythm, or more invasive monitoring, as needed
4. The potential to perform cardiopulmonary resuscitation (CPR) if required during the rewarming process
5. Minimal need for movement of the patient because of the propensity of movement to precipitate cardiac arrhythmias
6. Avoidance of thermal injury to skin

7. Avoidance of peripheral vasodilatation by keeping skin temperature modest
8. The ability to perform hemodialysis in the case of poisoning, e.g., barbiturates, while treatment for hypothermia is underway
9. An efficient, controllable means of heat delivery.

In considering the above characteristics, and extrapolating from our hyperthermia experience, we concluded that radiant heat rewarming might represent an optimal approach. It should be again pointed out that the transfer of radiant heat is far more efficient than conductive heating since radiant heat exchange is a fourth power function (Law and Pettigrew 1980; Robins et al. 1983b; Houdas and Ring 1982). After a positive experience using a hypothermic porcine model (Robins et al., unpublished), we have utilized a radiant heat approach to rewarming human exposure victims (Robins et al., unpublished). As part of this experience with two victims, we were able to unexpectedly salvage severely frostbitten limbs. This positive experience may relate to avoidance of high body surface temperature and hence thermal injury. This may represent a significant factor in the treatment of frostbite, not fully recognized by trauma physicians. In this regard, Herman et al. (1984b) has experimentally shown that cells climatized to low temperatures will be thermally injured at temperatures significantly lower than is the case when they are cultured at 37 °C.
In summary, the above discussion is meant to highlight an area of medical practice in which research derived from hyperthermic oncology may be relevant.

7.1.3 Acquired Immunodeficiency Syndrome

As discussed previously, many have been interested in the potential of treating retroviruses with 42 °C WBH (Macy and Gasper 1988; Yatvin 1988; Weatherburn 1988). In this regard, human immunodeficiency virus (HIV), the etiological cause of acquired immunodeficiency syndrome (AIDS), is a retrovirus of the family *Lentivirinae* (Sonigo et al. 1985). It is important to recognize that the HIV genome carries a reverse transcriptase. This enzyme catalyzes the synthesis of cDNA from the viral DNA. The cDNA can then integrate itself into the chromosomal DNA of the infected cell. The relevance of these aspects of AIDS to hyperthermia will become apparent in the discussion to follow.
Weatherburn suggested WBH as a general therapy for AIDS and its sequela. Yatvin (1988) hypothesized an approach to AIDS using hyperthermia along with anesthetics, dietary modification, or hydrophobic compounds such as butylated hydroxytoluene and adamantine, either alone or in combination. Clearly, *preclinical* research investigating the effects of hyperthermia in combination with other agents to attack the viral envelope might be warranted and could lead to interesting results.
A careful review of the available information relative to AIDS and the use of WBH, however, does not justify the empiric *clinical* use of WBH for this syndrome. Due to the devastating nature of AIDS many are predisposed to seek out panacea cures. Interesting media reports (USA) suggested that a patient treated with WBH had experienced reconstitution of his immune system, a complete remission of his Kaposi's sarcoma (KS) and improvement in virological parameters. A site visiting team from the Division of AIDS, the National Institute of Allergy and Infectious Disease, headed by the Chief of the Community Clinical Research Branch could find no objective evidence for these claims.
In spite of the lack of validation for the reported claim of a total remission of an AIDS patient treated with WBH, it is instructive to examine the potential scientific basis for observing the claimed result. The three positive phenomena reported, i.e., rapid restoration of the patient's immune status, prompt remission of the KS, and elimination of the HIV virus – would logically have required three independent hyperthermia-related mechanisms. The simultaneous reversal of these three remotely interrelated measures of this complex syndrome would, of course, represent an unusual coincidence if true.
In examining each aspect of this case, the following observations may be pertinent. Upon pathological review, the patient's pretreatment diagnosis of KS could not be confirmed. Further, as has been pointed out earlier in this text, WBH remissions of neoplastic processes are exceedingly short and invariably never complete (Robins et al. 1984b). (Indeed, this is the basis for the position whereby WBH is used as an adjunct to other therapeutic modalities.)
With regard to improvement of a patient's immune system, as previously reviewed, WBH at 42 °C is not stimulatory; at best the only clinical data which suggest even a marginal immune stimulation have been obtained using a low temperature range (39.5 °–40.5 °C) (Robins et al. 1989b).
With regard to heat inactivation of HIV, it should be noted that although this is a relatively heat-sensitive virus, HIV strains are not sterilized in the temperature range of systemic hyperthermia (Spire et al. 1985; McDougal et al. 1985; Resnick et al. 1986; Martin et al. 1985). Clearly, if one were to attempt elimination of the virus, an approach whereby the entire host is

heated would be necessary. Beyond this, if one wishes to use heat to sensitize the virus to drugs, as suggested by Yatvin (1988), the fact that HIV is incorporated into the human DNA genome probably makes the virus totally resistant to heat inactivation (regardless of the addition of a sensitizer).

Finally, in concluding this section on the potential use of WBH in the treatment of AIDS, AIDS-related complex, or an anti-HIV antibody positive state, the relative contraindications to this clinical approach should be discussed. We have previously highlighted the activation of herpes simplex 1 (see Chap. 5) by WBH. Beyond this it has been shown by Geelen et al. (1987) that heat shock is capable of the transcriptional activation of the major intermediate early transcriptional unit of human cytomegalovirus. Moreover, Stanley and Bressler (1990) made several disturbing observations in studying the ability of heat shock to induce HIV expression from U1 and ACH-2 cells. Cells (U1) exposed to 41.9 °C for 2 h – followed by subculture at 37 °C – expressed increased levels of HIV compared to control cells. Consistent with this, reverse transcriptase was increased threefold by hyperthermic treatment of 41.8 °–42 °C for 2–3 h. Incubations of 39 °C, 40 °C, and 41 °C for up to 12 h caused no increase in reverse transcriptase activity; heating up to 42.7 °C, however, caused up to a four- to sixfold increase in both UI and ACH-2 cells. These researchers further demonstrated that these increases were associated with a marked increase in HIV RNA, and that virus particles so induced were fully infective.

Parenthetically, it should be noted that various cytokines (TNF-α, granulocyte-macrophage colony-stimulating factor (GM-CSF) and IL-6) can induce HIV production in U1 cells (Poli et al. 1990; Folks et al. 1987) and these cytokines can be induced by low-grade fever (Beutler and Cerami 1987; Gauldie et al. 1987; Mizel 1989; Stanley et al. 1990). Stanley and Bressler (1990) investigated the ability of physiological heat (40.5 °C) and cytokines to synergistically stimulate HIV induction. GM-CSF and IL-6 have been found to synergize with heat exposure to produce 8- and 16-fold increases in reverse transcriptase activity respectively. (Heat has not been found to have an effect on TNF-α, phorbol mystrate acetate (PMA) or IL-1β induction of reverse transcriptase.)

A variety of mechanisms for heat induction of HIV are possible. These range from the utilization of heat shock proteins by the viral replication system (Schlessinger 1986; Stanley and Bressler 1990) to direct induction of HIV transcription. Additionally the findings relative to cytokines described above may be relevant. Regardless of the mechanism involved, we believe that the aforementioned research and considerations are sufficient to confine current hyperthermia-AIDS related research to preclinical investigations.

7.2 Implications of WBH Research for General Medical Practice

We have previously described and discussed the biophysical changes which occur with WBH. Clearly, many of these changes as well as observations from the WBH suite and oncological hyperthermia research are relevant to other facets of medicine. In the preceding section on AIDS, as well as the earlier section on endocrine function, we reviewed the hormonal and cytokine changes associated with fever. Although the physiological implications of these observations to the febrile patient are clear, the relevancy of other aspects of WBH physiology may not be as obvious. A great deal of appropriate concern is invariably directed at the increase in heart rate which occurs with 41.8 °C WBH. Parenthetically, blocking this physiological response with β-blocker, e.g., propranolol, is contraindicated as it results in cardiovascular collapse (Robins et al. 1991 a). Hence, to avoid the risk of myocardial infarction and cardiac decompensation in patients undergoing WBH, patients must be prescreened for organic heart disease. What is not fully appreciated, however, which can be derived from WBH research, is that the relationship of core temperature to heart rate is not linear, and heart rate can become maximal at relatively low temperatures (39.5 °–40.5 °C). This observation is illustrated in Fig. 14, Chap. 5. Thus, it is our contention that fevers in elderly patients (at risk for coronary artery disease) should be addressed promptly, and that supplemental oxygen during a febrile episode may be appropriate. Further, patients undergoing immunotherapy (in which febrile episodes are common and are associated with significant alterations in fluid balance) might also be appropriately prescreened for organic heart disease.

Based upon our experience with WBH patients, it also appears that procedures often used in dealing with hospitalized febrile patients may not be appropriate. Specifically, it is clear that to maximize cooling of a WBH patient, one merely needs to allow for evaporative heat losses while maintaining intravenous support, as well as minimizing covering to optimize radiant heat losses, as discussed in the section on thermal regulation. Clearly wiping perspiration off a seriously febrile patient is contraindicated. In addition, placing of ice packs in the axilla of patients, covering the head with cold compresses, covering the patient both above and below with cooling blankets, and covering patients with blankets appear to make little physiological sense. Again, it should be stressed that radiant heat losses and evaporative heat losses are far more efficient than conductive losses. Supportive measures for febrile patients such as fluids, oxygen, or even transfusions to correct significant anemia are often neglected as are simple interventions to maximize exposed surface area.

7.3 Systemic Hyperthermia: Summary Reflections Regarding Neoplastic Disease

In the preceding text, we have selected various topics to highlight both for investigators in the field, as well as those who would wish to enter or evaluate this exciting new arena of research. We felt it was beyond the scope of this text to reiterate our previous reviews of therapeutic strategies involving WBH. Such outlines are readily available with regard to several focused topics, e.g., the use and rationale for systemic hyperthermia in treating intracranial neoplasms (Cohen et al. 1990); the use and rationale for combining intraperitoneal carboplatin and WBH in the treatment of ovarian cancer (Cohen and Robins 1990a); the use of WBH in the adjuvant setting (Robins 1984); and the use of WBH in the setting of BMT and/or leukemia (Robins et al. 1984a, b; 1986b; 1988c).

Implicit in the utility of systemic hyperthermia for neoplastic diseases is its use in the treatment of large-volume, deep-seated neoplasms. It is significant to recognize that although regional equipment has this same potential, treatment volumes remain a problem with regard to temperature homogeneity and stability. Additionally, local and regional technology is inadequate to heat the lungs (Bleehan and Cox 1985). WBH is the only approach to heating pulmonary disease currently (Robins et al. 1986a, 1988b). Contrary to the intuitive notion of many, breathing represents an extremely inefficient means of dissipating heat. The panting dog cannot dissipate heat, if evaporative heat losses from the tongue are prevented by preadministration with atropine to prevent salvation. Thus, the observations of Hugander et al. (1987) and Thrall et al. (1986) demonstrating that the temperature of the lung (an extremely vascular organ) closely approximates core temperature – should be expected.

In conclusion, although systemic hyperthermia has been added to the therapeutic armamentarium of several major cancer centers, further preclinical and clinical research is still required to establish the boundaries of its clinical utility. Clearly, the number of methodologies currently being used reflects a lack of consensus as to the optimal application of physiological and therapeutic principles to systemic hyperthermia. It is our current prejudice that future clinical trials demonstrating efficacy via phase III clinical studies will be requisite for the field to expand. The need for a cost-effective system for multiinstitutional trials is obvious. Inherent in any medical consideration of cost versus benefit must be a consideration of clinical toxicity.

Over two thousand years have passed since physicians intuitively approached fever as being therapeutically beneficial. Induced systemic hyperthermia has been studied for at least a century. During the past 20 years an unequivocal laboratory data base has been established in support of the use of systemic hyperthermia. In the next decade it is the task of investigative proponents of WBH to extend and extrapolate both laboratory and clinical research efforts to obtain definitive results in the context of randomized prospective clinical trials.

References

Adams GE, Stratford IJ, Rajaratnam S (1982) Interaction of the cytotoxic and sensitizing effects of electron-affinic drugs and hyperthermia. NCI Monogr 61:27–35

Adamson IYR, Young L, Orr FW (1987) Tumor metastasis after hyperoxic injury and repair of the pulmonary endothelium. Lab Invest 57:71–77

Adwankar MK, Chitnis MP (1984) Effect of hyperthermia alone and in combination with anticancer drugs on the viability of P388 leukemic cells. Tumori 70:231–234

Alberts DS, Peng YM, Chen HSG, Moon TE, Cetas TC, Hoschele JD (1980) Therapeutic synergism of hyperthermia-cis-platinum in a mouse tumor model. JNCI 65:455–461

Anderson RL, Ahier RG, Littleton JM (1983) Observasions on the cellular effects of ethanol and hyperthermia in vivo. Radiat Res 94:318–325

Ando K, Urano M, Kenton L, Kahn J (1987) Effect of thermochemotherapy on the development of spontaneous lung metastases. Int J Hyperthermia 3(5):453–458

Arcangeli G, Cevidalli A, Nervi C, Creton G (1983) Tumor control and therapeutic gain with different schedules of combined radiotherapy and local external hyperthermia in human cancer. Int J Radiat Oncol Biol Phys 9:1124–1134

Aristizabal SA, Oleson JR (1984) Combined interstitial irradiation and localized current field hyperthermia: results and conclusions from clinical studies. Cancer Res 44:4757s–4760s

Ashman RB, Nahmias AJ (1977) Enhancement of human lymphocyte responses to phytomitogens in vitro by incubation at elevated temperatures. Clin Asp Immunol 29:464–467

Atkinson ER (1979) Assessment of current hyperthermia technology. Cancer Res 39:2313–2324

Azocar J, Yunis EJ, Essex M (1982) Sensitivity of human natural killer cells to hyperthermia. Lancet 1:16–17

Baba H, Siddik ZH, Strebel FR, Jenkins GN, Bull JMC (1989) Increased therapeutic gain of combined cis-diamminedichloroplatinum (II) and whole body hyperthermia therapy by optimal heat/drug scheduling. Cancer Res 49:7041–7044

Baker HW, Snedecor PA, Goss JC, Galen WP, Gallucci JJ, Horowitz IJ, Dugan K (1982) Regional hyperthermia for cancer. Am J Surg 143:586–590

Barlogie B, Corry PM, Yip E, Lippmann L, Johnston DA, Khalil K, Tenzynski TF, Reilly E, Lawson R, Dosik G, Rigor B, Hankenson R, Freireich EJ (1979) Total-body hyperthermia with and without chemotherapy for advanced human neoplasms. Cancer Res 39:1481–1489

Barlogie B, Corry PM, Drewinko B (1980) In vitro thermochemotherapy of human colon cancer cells with cis-dichlorodiamineplatinum(II) and mitomycin C. Cancer Res 40:1165–1166

Barranco SC, Novak JK, Humphrey RM (1975) Studies on recovery from chemically induced damage in mammalian cells. Cancer Res 35:1194–1204

Bates DA, MacKillop WJ (1989) The effect of hyperthermia on the uptake and cytotoxicity of melphalan in Chinese hamster ovary cells. Int J Radiat Oncol Biol Phys 16:187–191

Beckley SA, Madajewicz S, Higby P, Takita H, Bhargava A, Wajsman Z, Pontes JE (1982) Combination of systemic hyperthermia with chemotherapy. Proc Am Soc Clin Oncol 23:116 (abstract)

Bell CL, Yocum D, Blank J, Taylor CA (1983) Malignant hyperthermia: association with the HLA antigens A11, B35 and C4. In: Lomax P, Schonbaum E (eds) Environment, drugs, and thermoregulation. Karger, Basel, p 164

Belli JA, Bonte FJ (1963) Influence of temperature on the radiation response of mammalian cells in tissue culture. Radiat Res 18:272–276

Ben-Hur E, Elkind MM (1974) Thermally enhanced radioresponse of cultured Chinese hamster cells: damage and repair of single-stranded DNA and a DNA complex. Radiat Res 59:484–495

Ben-Hur E, Bronk BV, Elkind MM (1972) Thermally enhanced radiosensitivity of cultured Chinese hamster cells. Nature New Biol 238:209–210

Ben-Hur E, Elkind MM, Bronk BV (1974) Thermally enhanced radioresponse of cultured Chinese hamster cells: inhibition of repair of sublethal damage and enhancement of lethal damage. Radiat Res 58:38–51

Berenbaum MC, Fluck PA, Hurst NP (1973) Depression of lymphocyte responses after surgical trauma. Br J Exp Pathol 54:597–607

Beutler B, Cerami A (1987) Cachectin: more than a tumor necrosis factor. N Engl J Med 316:379

Bigelow WG, Hopps JA, Callaghan JC (1952) Radio frequency rewarming in resuscitation from severe hypothermia. Can J Med Sci 30:185–193

Bitran JD, Desser RK, Shapiro CM, Michel A, Kozloff MF, Billings AA (1983) Response to secondary therapy in patients with adenocarcinoma of the breast previously treated with adjuvant chemotherapy. Cancer 51:381–384

Blair RM, Levin W (1978) Clinical experience of the induction and maintenance of whole-body hyperthermia. In: Streffer C, Beuningen D, Dietzel F et al. (eds) Cancer therapy by hyperthermia and radiation. Urban and Schwarzenberg, Baltimore, pp 318–321

Blair E, Swan H, Virtue R (1977) Clinical hypothermia: a study of ice water surface immersion and shortwave diathermy techniques. Ann Surg 22:574–577

Bleehan NM, Cox JD (1985) Radiotherapy for lung cancer. Int J Radiat Oncol Biol Phys 11:1001–1007

Bonadonna G, Valagussa P (1981) Dose-response effect of adjuvant chemotherapy in breast cancer. N Engl J Med 304:10–15

Bork-Wolwer L, Buhring M, Krippner H (1978) T-lymphocytopenia during standardized hyperthermia. In: Streffer C (ed) Proceedings of the 2nd symposium on cancer therapy by hyperthermia and radiation. Urban and Schwarzenberg, Baltimore, p 306–308

Bowden GT, Kasunic MD (1981) Hyperthermic potentiation of the effects of a clinically significant x-ray dose on survival, DNA damage, and DNA repair. Radiat Res 87:109–120

Bowman W (1977) Medical aspects of mountain climbing. J Winter Emerg Care 2:31–47

Braun J, Hahn GM (1975) Enhanced cell killing by bleomycin and 43 °C hyperthermia and the inhibition of recovery from potentially lethal damage. Cancer Res 35:2921–2927

Brett DE, Schloerb PR (1962) Intermittent hyperthermia on Walker 256 carcinoma. Arch Surg 85:154–157

Brewer JA, Hank JA, Wendel T, Schmeling GJ, Blank JL, Morrissey LW, Robins HI, Sondel PM (1983) Heated lymphocytes express HLA-DR antigens despite their inability to stimulate in MLC. Tissue Antigens 22:246–256

Bromer RH, Mitchell JB, Soares N (1982) Response of human hematopoietic precursor cells (CFUc) to hyperthermia and radiation. Cancer Res 42:1261–1265

Bronk BV, Wilkins RJ, Regan JD (1973) Thermal enhancement of DNA damage by an alkylating agent in human cells. Biochem Biophys Res Commun 52:1064–1070

Brownlie SA, Campbell JG, Head KW, Iailah P, McTaggart HS, McVie JG (1978) Prednisolone treatment of hereditary pig lymphoma. Eur J Cancer 14:983–994

Bruns P (1888) Die heilwirkung des erysipeln auf geschwülste. In: Bruns P (ed) Beiträge zur klinischen chirurgie. Mittheilungen aus der chirurgischen Klinik zu Tübingen, vol 3. Laupp, Tübingen, pp 443–446

Bull JM, Lees D, Schuette W, Whang-Peng J, Smith R, Byrnum G, Atkinson R, Gottdiener J, Gralnick HR, Shawker TH, DeVita V (1979a) Whole body hyperthermia: a Phase I trial of potential adjuvant chemotherapy. Ann Intern Med 90:317–323

Bull JM, Whang-Peng J, Lees DE, Smith R, Schuette W, Kim YD, DeVita VT (1979b) A Phase I trial of systemic heat and adriamycin. Proc Am Soc Clin Oncol 20:398

Bull JM, Lees D, Schuette WH, Smith R, Glatstein E, DeVita VT (1982) Immunological and physiological responses to whole-body hyperthermia. NCI Monogr 61:177–181

Burmeister P, Neumann H, Fabricius H, Engelhardt R (1980) Endocrine changes in whole body hyperthermia. In: Dethlefson LA (ed) Proceedings of the 3rd international symposium on cancer therapy by hyperthermia, drugs and radiation. Colorado State University, Ft Collins, Colorado, p 85

Busch W (1866) Über den Einfluß welche heftigere erysipeln zuweilig auf organisierte Neubildungen ausüben. Verh Naturhist Preuss Rhein Westphal 23:28–30

Cabanac M (1975) Temperature regulation. Annu Rev Physiol 37:415–438

Calvert AH, Harland SJ, Newell DR, Siddik ZH, Jones AC, Mcelwain TJ, Raju S, Wiltshaw E, Smith IE, Baker JM, Peckham MJ, Harrap KR (1982) Early clinical studies with cis-diammine-1,1-cyclobutane dicarboxylate platinum II. Cancer Chemother Pharmacol 9:140–147

Cater DB, Silver IA, Watkinson DA (1964) Combined therapy with 220 kV roentgen and 10 cm microwave heating in rat hepatoma. Acta Radiol 2:321–336

Cavaliere R, Giocatto EC, Giovanella BC, Heidelberger C, Johonson RO, Margottini RM, Mondovi B, Moricca G, Rassifanell A (1967) Selective heat sensitivity of cancer cells. Cancer 20:1351–1381

Chadwick KH, Leenhouts HP (1973) A molecular theory of cell survival. Phys Med Biol 18:78–87

Chen TT, Heidelberger C (1969) Quantitative studies on the malignant transformation of mouse prostate cells by carcinogenic hydrocarbons in vitro. Int J Cancer 4:166–178

Chlebowski RT, Block JB, Cundiff D, Dietrich MF (1982) Doxorubicin cytotoxicity enhanced by local anaesthetics in a human melanoma cell line. Cancer Treat Rep 66:121–125

Clark A, Robins HI, Vorpahl JW, Yatvin MB (1983) Structural changes in murine cancer associated with hyperthermia and lidocaine. Cancer Res 43:1716–1723

Clark EP, Dewey WC, Lett JT (1981) Recovery of CHO cells from hyperthermic potentiation to x-rays: repair of DNA and chromatin. Radiat Res 85:302–313

Clawson RE, Egorin MJ, Fox BM, Ross LA, Bachur NR (1981) Hyperthermic modification of cyclophosphamide metabolism in rat microsomes and liver slices. Life Sci 28:1133–1137

Cohen JD, Robins HI (1987) Hyperthermic enhancement of cis-diammine-1,1-cyclobutane dicarboxylate platinum(II) cytotoxicity in human leukemia cells in vitro. Cancer Res 47:4335–4337

Cohen JD, Robins HI (1990a) Whole body hyperthermia and intraperitoneal carboplatin in residual ovarian cancer. In: Bicher HI, McLaren JR, Pigluicci G (eds) Consensus of hyperthermia for the 1990s; advances in medicine and biology series. Plenum, New York pp 197–202

Cohen JD, Robins HI (1990b) Thermal enhancement of tetraplatin and carboplatin cytotoxicity in human leukemic cells in vitro. Int J Hyperthermia 6:1013–1017

Cohen JD, Robins HI, Mulcahy RT, Gipp JJ, Bouck N (1988) Interactions between hyperthermia and irradiation in two human lymphoblastic leukemia cell lines in vitro. Cancer Res 48:3576–3580

Cohen JD, Robins HI, Schmitt CL (1989a) Interactions of hyperthermia with carboplatin, cisplatin, and etoposide in human leukemia cells in vitro. Cancer Lett 44:205–210

Cohen JD, Robins HI, Schmitt CL, Tanner M (1989b) Interactions of thymidine, hyperthermia, and cis-diammine-1,1-cyclobutane dicarboxylate platinum(II) in human T-cell leukemia. Cancer Res 49:5805–5809

Cohen JD, Robins HI, Javid MJ (1990) Sensitization of C6 glioma to carboplatin cytotoxicity by hyperthermia and thymidine. J Neurooncol 9:1–8

Coley WR (1893) The treatment of malignant tumors by repeated inoculations of erysipelas: with a report of ten original cases. Am J Sci 105:487–511

Collins FG, Skibba JL (1979) Effect of hyperthermia and mechlorethamine on hepatic function in isolated perfused liver. Proc Am Assoc Cancer Res 20:125

Collins FG, Skibba JL (1983) Altered hepatic functions and microsomal activity in perfused rat liver by hyperthermia combined with alkylating agents. Cancer Biochem Biophys 6:205–211

Collis M, Steinman A, Chaney R (1977) Accidental hypothermia: experimental study of practical rewarming methods. Aviat Space Environ Med 48:625–632

Corry PM, Frazier OH (1982) Methods for the induction of systemic hyperthermia. In: Nussbaum GH (ed) Physical aspects of hyperthermia. American Association of Physicists in medicine medical physics monograph, vol 8. American Institute of Physics, Inc., New York, NY, pp 587–599

Corry PM, Robinson S, Getz S (1977) Hyperthermic effects on DNA repair mechanisms. Radiology 123:457–482

Corry PM, Barlogia B, Telchen EJ, Armour EP (1982) Ultrasound-induced hyperthermia for the treatment of human superficial tumors. Int J Radiat Oncol Biol Phys 8:1225–1229

Corry PM, Jabboury K, Armour EP, Kong JS (1984) Human cancer treatment with ultrasound. IEEE Trans Sonics Ultrasound SU 31:444–456

Cronau LH, Bourke DL, Bull JM (1984) General anesthesia for whole body hyperthermia. Cancer Res 44 [suppl] 4873 s–4877 s

Dahl O (1983) Hyperthermic potentiation of doxorubicin and 4-epi-doxorubicin in a transplantable neurogenic rat tumor (BT4A) in BD IX rats. Int J Radiat Oncol Biol Phys 9:203–207

Dahl O, Mella O (1982) Enhanced effect of combined hyperthermia and chemotherapy (bleomycin, BCNU) in a neurogenic rat tumor (BT4A) in vivo. Anticancer Res 2:259–264

Dahl O, Mella O (1983) Effect of timing and sequence of hyperthermia and cyclophosphamide on a neurogenic rat tumor (BT4A) in vivo. Cancer 52:983–987

Dahl O, Mella O (1984) Timing and sequence of hyperthermia and drugs. Hyperthermic oncology, 1984, vol 1. Proceedings of the 4th international symposium on hyperthermic oncology, pp 425–428

De Horatius RJ, Hosea JM, Van Epps DE, Reed WP, Edwards WS, Williams RC Jr (1977) Immunologic function in humans before and after hyperthermia and chemotherapy for disseminated malignancy. JNCI 58:905–911

Delbruck HG, Allouche M, Jasmin C (1980) Influence of increased temperature on the inhibition of rat osteosarcoma cell multiplication in vitro by interferon. Biomedicine 33:239–241

De Silva V, Tofilon PJ, Gutin PH, Dewey WC, Buckley N, Deen DF (1985) Comparative study of the effects of hyperthermia and BCNU on BCNU-sensitive and BCNU-resistant 9L rat brain tumor cells. Radiat Res 103:363–372

Dewey WC (1979) In vitro systems: standardization of endpoints. Int J Radiat Oncol Biol Phys 5:1165–1174

Dewey WC (1984) Inactivation of mammalian cells by combined hyperthermia and radiation. Front Radiat Ther Oncol 18:29–40

Dewey WC, Westra A, Miller HH, Nagasawa H (1971) Heat-induced lethality and chromosomal damage in synchronized Chinese hamster cells treated with 5-bromodeoxyuridine. Int J Radiat Biol 20:505–520

Dewey WC, Hopwood LE, Sapareto SA, Gerweck LE (1977a) Cellular responses to combinations of hyperthermia and radiation. Radiology 123:463–474

Dewey WC, Thrall DE, Gillette EL (1977b) Hyperthermia and radiation – a selective thermal effect on chronically hypoxic tumor cells in vivo. Int J Radiat Oncol Biol Phys 2: 99–103

Dewey WC, Freeman ML, Raaphorst GP, Clark EP, Wong RS, Highfield DP, Spiro JS, Tomosovic SP, Denman DL, Coss RA (1980) Cell biology of hyperthermia and radiation. In: Meyn RA, Whiters HR (eds) Radiation biology in cancer research. Raven, New York, pp 489–621

Dewhirst MW, Sim DA (1984a) The utility of thermal dose as a predictor of tumor and normal tissue responses to combined radiation and hyperthermia. Cancer Res [Suppl] 44:4772s–4780s

Dewhirst MW, Sim DA (1984b) Analysis of prognostic variables which influence early and long-term response of pet animal tumors to radiation alone and radiation plus heat. Front Radiat Ther Oncol 18:47–55

Dewhirst MW, Connor WG, Sim DA (1982) Preliminary results of a Phase II trial of spontaneous animal tumors to heat and/or radiation: early normal tissue response and tumor volume influence on initial response. Int J Radiat Oncol Biol Phys 8:1951–1961

Dewhirst MW, Sim DA, Sapareto S, Connor WG (1984) The importance of minimum tumor temperature in determining early and long-term responses of spontaneous canine and feline tumors to heat and radiation. Cancer Res 44:43–50

Dewhirst MW, Winget JM, Edelstein-Keshet L, Sylvester J, Engler MJ, Thrall DE, Page RL, Oleson JR (1987) Clinical application of thermal isoeffect dose. Int J Hyperthermia 3:307–318

Dickson JA (1984) The abscopal response and tumor control in human cancer. In: Overgaard J (ed) Proceedings of the 4th international symposium on hyperthermia oncol. Taylor and Francis, London, pp 467–471

Dickson JA, Ellis HA (1974) Stimulation of tumour cell dissemination by raised temperature (42 °C) in rats with transplanted Yoshida tumours. Nature 248:354–358

Dickson JA, Muckle DS (1972) Total body hyperthermia versus primary tumour hyperthermia in the treatment of the rabbit VX2 carcinoma. Cancer Res 32:1916–1923

Dickson JA, Oswald BE (1976) The sensitivity of a malignant cell line to hyperthermia (42 °C) at low intracellular pH. Br J Cancer 34:262–271

Dickson JA, Shah SA (1977) Technology for the hyperthermic treatment of large solid tumours at 50 °C. Clin Oncol 3:301–318

Dickson JA, Shah SA (1982) Hyperthermia, the immune response and tumor metastasis. In: Dethlefsen L, Dewey WC (eds) Proceedings of the 3rd symposium on cancer therapy by hyperthermia, drug and radiation, Bethesda, MD. JNCI 61:183–192

Dickson JA, MacKenzie A, McLeod K (1979) Temperature gradients in pigs during whole body hyperthermia at 42 °C. J Appl Physiol Respir Environ Exercise Physiol 47:712

Dikomey E (1982) Effect of hyperthermia at 42° and 45 °C on repair of radiation-induced DNA strand breaks in CHO cells. Int J Radiat Biol 41:603–614

Dinarello CA (1985) An update on human interleukin-1: from molecular biology to clinical relevance. J Clin Immunol 5:287–297

Dinarello CA, Bernheim HA, Duff GW, Le HV, Nagabhushan TL, Hamilton NC, Coceani F (1984) Mechanisms of fever induced by recombinant human interferon. J Clin Invest 74:906–913

Dinarello CA, Dempsey RA, Allegretta M, LoPreste G, Dainiak N, Parkinson DR, Mier JW (1986) Inhibitory effects of elevated temperature on human cytokine production and natural killer activity. Cancer Res 46:6236–6241

Doan CA, Hargreaves MM, Kester L (1937) Differential reaction of bone marrow, connective tissue and lymph nodes to hyperpyrexia. In: Simpson WM, Bierman W (eds) Fever therapy. Hoeber, New York, pp 40–41

Donaldson SS, Gordon LF, Hahn GM (1978) Protective effect of hyperthermia against the cytotoxicity of actinomycin D on Chinese hamster cells. Cancer Treat Rep 62:1489–1495

Douglas MA, Parks LC, Begin J (1981) Sudden myelopathy secondary to therapeutic total body hyperthermia after spinal cord irradiation. N Engl J Med 304:583–585

Douple EB, Strohbehn JW, de Sieyes DC, Alborough DP, Trembly BS (1982) Therapeutic potentiation of cis-diammineplatinum(II) and radiation by interstitial microwave hyperthermia in a mouse tumor. NCI Monogr 61:259–262

Downing JF, Taylor MW (1987) The effect of in vivo hyperthermia on selected lymphokines in man. Lymphokine Res 6:103–109

Dubois M, Sato S, Lees DW, Bull JM, Smith R, White BG, Moore H, MacNamara TE (1980) Electroencephalographic changes during whole body hyperthermia in humans. Electroencephalogr Clin Neurophysiol 50:486

Duff WG, Durum SK (1982) Fever and immunoregulation: hyperthermia, interleukins 1 and 2, and T-cell proliferation. Yale J Biol Med 55:437–442

Dugle DL, Gillespie CJ, Chapman JE (1976) DNA strand breaks, repair, and survival in x-irradiated mammalian cells. Proc Natl Acad Sci USA 73:809–812

Engelhardt R (1984) Whole-body-hyperthermia methods and clinical results. In: Overgaard J (ed) Hyperthermic oncology, vol 2. Taylor and Francis, Philadelphia, pp 263–277

Engelhardt R (1987) Hyperthermia and drugs. In: Streffer C (ed) Hyperthermia and the therapy of malignant tumors. Springer, Berlin Heidelberg New York, pp 136–203 (Recent results in cancer research, vol 104)

Engelhardt R (1988) Summary of recent clinical experience in whole-body hyperthermia combined with chemotherapy. In: Issels RD, Wilmanns W (eds) Application of hyperthermia in the treatment of cancer. Springer, Berlin Heidelberg New York, pp 200–204 (Recent Results in cancer research, vol 107)

Engelhardt R, Muller U, Weth-Simon R, Neumann HA, Lohr GW (1990) Treatment of disseminated malignant melanoma with cisplatin in combination with whole-body hyperthermia and doxorubicin. Int J Hyperthermia 6:511–515

Euler-Rolle J, Priesching A, Vormittag E, Tschakaloff C, Polterauer P (1978) Prevention of cardiac complications during whole-body hyperthermia by beta receptor blockage. In: Streffer C, van Beuningen D, Dietzel F (eds) Cancer therapy by hyperthermia and radiation. Urban and Schwarzenberg, Baltimore, pp 302–305

Fabricius HA, Stahn R, Metzger B, Fluck K, Engelhardt R, Neumann H, Sellin D (1978) Changes in cellular immunological functions of healthy adults induced by a one-hour 40 °C hyperthermia. In: Streffer et al. (eds) Proceedings of the 2nd international symposium on cancer therapy by hyperthermia and radiation. Urban and Schwarzenberg, Baltimore, pp 309–311

Faithfull NS, Reinhold HS, Berg AP, van Rhoon GC, Van der Zee J, Wike-Hooley JL (1984) Cardiovascular changes during whole-body treatment of advanced malignancy. Eur J Appl Physiol 53:274–281

Faithfull NS, Vandenberg AP, Van Rhoon GC (1982) Cardiovascular and oxygenation changes during whole body hyperthermia. Adv Exp Med Biol 157:57

Fernandez JP, O'Rourke RA, Ewy GA (1970) Rapid active external rewarming in accidental hypothermia. J Am Med Assoc 212:153–156

Fidler IJ (1978) Tumor heterogeneity and the biology of cancer invasion and metastases. Cancer Res 38:2651–2660

Fisher GA, Hahn GM (1982) Enhancement of cisdiaminedichloroplatinum (cis-DDP) cytotoxicity by hyperthermia. NCI Monogr 61:255–257

Folks TM, Justement J, Kinter A, Dinarello CA, Fauci AS (1987) Cytokine-induced expression of HIV-1 in a chronically infected promonocytic cell line. Science 238:800

Freeman ML, Dewey WC, Hopwood LE (1977) Effect of pH on hyperthermia cell survival. JNCI 58:1837–1839

Freeman ML, Holahan EV, Highfield DP, Raaphorst GP, Spiro IJ, Dewey WC (1981) The effect of pH on hyperthermic and x-ray induced cell killing. Int J Radiat Oncol Biol Phys 7:211–216

Fujiwara K, Kohno I, Miyao J, Sekiba K (1984) The effect of heat on cell proliferation and the uptake of anti-cancer drugs into tumour. Proceedings of the 4th international symposium on hyperthermic oncology, pp 405–408

Galant EM, Ahern CP (1983) Malignant hyperthermia: responses of skeletal muscles to general anesthetics. Mayo Clin Proc 58:758

Gauldie J, Richards C, Harnish D, Lansdorp P, Baumann H (1987) Interferon β_2/B-cell stimulatory factor type 2 shares identity with monocyte-derived hepatocyte-stimulating factor and regulates the major acute phase protein response in liver cells. Proc Natl Acad Sci USA 84:7251

Gee AP, Williams AE, Pettigrew RT, Smith AN (1978) Effects of whole body hyperthermia therapy on the general immunocompetence of the advanced cancer patient. In: Streffer et al. (eds) Proceedings of the 2nd international symposium on cancer therapy by hyperthermia and radiation. Urban and Schwarzenberg, Baltimore, pp 312–315

Geelen JLMC, Boom R, Klaver GPM, Minnaar M, Feltkamp CW, Van Milligen FJ, Sol CJA, Van der Noordaa J (1987) Transcriptional activation of the major immediate early transcription unit of human cytomegalovirus by heat-shock, arsenite and protein synthesis inhibitors. J Gen Virol 68: 2925

Gerad H, Egorin MJ, Whitacre M, Van Echo DA, Aisner J (1983) Renal failure and platinum pharmacokinetics in three patients treated with cis-diamminedichloroplatinum (II) and whole body hyperthermia. Cancer Chemother Pharmacol 11:162–166

Gerad H, Van Echo DA, Whitacre M, Ashman M, Helrich M, Foy J, Ostrow S, Wiernik PH, Aisner J (1984) Doxorubicin, cyclophosphamide, and whole body hyperthermia for treatment of advanced soft tissue sarcoma. Cancer 53:2585–2591

Gerweck LE (1982) Effect of microenvironmental factors on the response of cells to single and fractionated heat treatments. NCI Monogr 61:19–26

Gerweck LE, Rottinger E (1976) Enhancement of mammalian cell sensitivity to hyperthermia by pH alteration. Radiat Res 67:508–511

Gerweck LE, Gillette EL, Dewey WC (1974) Killing of Chinese hamster cells in vitro by heat under hypoxic or aerobic conditions. Eur J Cancer 10:691–693

Gerweck LE, Gillette EL, Dewey WC (1975) Effect of heat and radiation on synchronous Chinese hamster cells: killing and repair. Radiat Res 64:611–623

Ghussen F, Nagel K, Groth W, Muller JM, Stutzer H (1984) A prospective randomized study of regional extremity perfusion in patients with malignant melanoma. Ann Surg 200:764–768

Gillette EL, Ensley BA (1979) Effect of heating order on radiation response of mouse tumor and skin. Int J Radiat Oncol Biol Phys 5:209–213

Girard DJ, Fleischaker RJ, Sinskey AJ (1982) Kinetics of human beta interferon production under different temperature conditions. Interferon Res 2:471–477

Giovanella BD, Morgan AC, Stehlin JS, Williams LJ (1973) Selective lethal effect of supranormal temperatures on mouse sarcoma cells. Cancer Res 33:2568–2578

Goffinet DR, Choi KY, Martin Brown J (1977) The combined effects of hyperthermia and ionizing radiation on the adult mouse spinal cord. Radiat Res 72:238–245

Goldenberg DM, Langner M (1971) Direct and abscopal antitumor action of local hyperthermia. Z Naturforsch 26b:359–361

Golden F (1972) Accidental hypothermia. JR Nav Med Serv 58:196–206

Goldin EM, Leeper DB (1981) The effect of low pH on thermotolerance induction using fractionated 45 °C hyperthermia. Radiat Res 85:472–479

Goss P, Parsons PG (1977) The effect of hyperthermia and melphalan on survival of human fibroblast strains and melanoma cell lines. Cancer Res 37:152–156

Gregory R, Doolittle W (1973) Accidental hypothermia: part II. Clinical implications of experimental studies. Alaska Med 15:48–52

Gregory RT, Patton JF, McFadden JT (1973) Cardiovascular effects of arteriovenous shunt rewarming following experimental hypothermia. Surgery 73:561–571

Grogan JB, Parks LC, Minaberry D (1980) Polymorphonuclear leukocyte function in cancer patients treated with total body hyperthermia. Cancer 45:2611–2615

Groveman DS, Borden EC, Merritt JA, Robins HI, Steeves RA,

Bryan GT (1984) Augmented antiproliferative effects of interferons at elevated temperatures. Cancer Res 44:5517–5521

Guillemin R, Vargo T, Rossier J, Minick S, Ling N, Rivier C, Vale W, Bloom F (1977) β-Endorphin and adrenocorticotropin are secreted concomitantly by the pituitary gland. Science, 197; 1367–1368

Guntupalli KK, Sladen A (1982) Induced total body hyperthermia: a comparison of pre- and post-treatment physiological parameters. Crit Care Med 10:220 (abstract)

Guntupalli KK, Sladen A, Selker GR, Weinstock E, Wilks E, Wilks DH, Passmore J, Guntupalli SJ (1984) Effects of induced total-body hyperthermia on phosphorus metabolism in humans. Am J Med 77:250–254

Haas GP, Klugo RC, Hetzel FW, Barton EE, Cernyl IC (1984) The synergistic effect of hyperthermia and chemotherapy on murine transitional cell carcinoma. J Urol 132:828–833

Habu S, Fukui H, Shimamwa K, Kasai M, Nagi Y, Okumura K, Tamaoki N (1981) In vivo effects of anti-asialo GM_1. Reduction of NK activity and enhancement of tumor growth in nude mice. J Immunol 127:34–39

Hahn GM (1974) Metabolic aspects of the role of hyperthermia in mammalian cell inactivation and their possible relevance to cancer treatment. Cancer Res 34:3117–3123

Hahn GM (1978) Interactions of drugs and hyperthermia in vitro and in vivo. In: Streffer C, Van Beuningen D, Dietzel F, Toettinger E, Robinson JE, Scherer E, Seeber S, Trott KD (eds) Cancer therapy by hyperthermia and radiation. Proceedings of the 2nd international symposium, June 2–4, 1977, Essen. Urban and Scharzenberg, Baltimore, pp 72–79

Hahn GM (1979) Potential for therapy of drugs and hyperthermia. Cancer Res 39:2264–2268

Hahn GM (1982) Hyperthermia and cancer. Plenum, New York

Hahn GM (1983) Hyperthermia to enhance drug delivery. In: Chabner BA (ed) Rational basis for chemotherapy, UCLA symposia on molecular and cellular biology, vol 4. UCLA symposium on the rational basis for chemotherapy, Keystone, CO, 1982. Liss, New York, pp 427–436

Hahn GM, Li GC (1982) Interactions of hyperthermia and drugs. Treatments and probes. NCI Monogr 61:317–323

Hahn GM, Shiu EC (1983) Effect of pH and elevated temperature on the cytotoxicity of some chemotherapeutic agents in Chinese hamster cells in vitro. Cancer Res 43:5789–5791

Hahn GM, Shiu EC (1986) Adaptation to low pH modifies thermal and thermo-chemical responses of mammalian cells. Int J Hyperthermia 2:379–387

Hahn GM, Strande DP (1976) Cytotoxic effects of hyperthermia and adriamycin on Chinese hamster cells. JNCI 57:1063–1067

Hahn GM, Braun J, Har-Kedar I (1975) Thermochemotherapy: synergism between hyperthermia (42°–43 °C) and adriamycin (or bleomycin) in mammalian cell inactivation (cancer chemotherapy/cell membranes). Proc Natl Acad Sci USA 72:937–940

Hahn GM, Li GC, Shue E (1977) Interaction of amphotericin B and 43 °C hyperthermia. Cancer Res 37:761–764

Hank JA, Brewer JA, Brown LR, Reitnauer PJ, Robins HI, Sondel P (1983) Differential effect of heating on autologous versus allogeneic MLC stimulation by Epstein Barr virus (EBV) transformed LCL cells (abstract). Proceedings of the 5th international congress of immunology, Kyoto, Japan, no 508–520

Hanna N (1982) Inhibition of experimental tumor metastasis by selective activation of natural killer cells. Cancer Res 42:1337–1342

Hanson DF, Murphy PA, Silicano R, Shin HS (1983) The effect of temperature on the activation of thymocytes by interleukin 1 and 2. J Immunol 130 (1):216–221

Harari PM, Fuller DJM, Carper SW, Croghan MK, Meyskens FL, Shimm DS, Gerner EW (1990) Polyamine biosynthesis inhibitors combined with systemic hyperthermia in cancer therapy. Int J Radiat Oncol Biol Phys 19:89–96

Harisiadis L, Hall EJ, Karljevic U, Borek C (1975) Hyperthermia: biological studies at the cellular level. Radiology 117:447–452

Hassanzadeh M, Chapman IV (1983) Thermal enhancement of bleomycin-induced tumor growth delay: the effect of dose fractionation. Eur J Cancer Clin Oncol 19:1517–1519

Hayward JS, Steinman AM (1975) Accidental hypothermia: an experimental study of inhalation rewarming. Aviat Space Environ Med 46:1236–1240

Hazan G, Ben-Hur E, Yerushalmi A (1981) Synergism between hyperthermia and cyclophosphamide in vivo: the effect of dose fractionation. Eur J Cancer 17:681–684

Hazan G, Lurie H, Yerushalmi A (1984) Sensitization of combined cis-platinum and cyclophosphamide by local hyperthermia in mice bearing the Lewis lung carcinoma. Oncology 41:68–69

Henle KJ, Dethlefsen LA (1978) Heat fractionation and thermotolerance: a review. Cancer Res 38:1843–1851

Henle KJ, Leeper DB (1976) Combinations of hyperthermia (40°, 45 °C) with radiation. Radiology 121:451–454

Herman TS (1983a) Effect of temperature on the cytotoxicity of vindesine, amsacrine, and mitoxantrone. Cancer Treat Rep 67:1019–1022

Herman TS (1983b) Temperature dependence of adriamycin, cis-diamminedichloroplatinum, bleomycin, and 1,3-bis(2-chloroethyl)-1-nitrosourea cytotoxicity in vitro. Cancer Res 43:517–520

Herman TS, Cress AE, Sweets C, Gerner EW (1981) Reversal of resistance to methotrexate by hyperthermia in Chinese hamster ovary cells. Cancer Res 41:3840–3843

Herman TS, Sweets CC, White DM, Gerner EW (1982a) Effect of heating on lethality due to hyperthermia and selected chemotherapeutic drugs. JNCI 68:487–491

Herman TS, Zukoski CS, Anderson RM (1982b) Review of the current status of whole body hyperthermia administered by water circulation techniques. NCI Monogr 61:365

Herman TS, Zukoski CS, Anderson RM, Hutter JJ, Blitt CD, Malone JM, Larson DF, Dean JC, Roth HB (1982c) Whole-body hyperthermia and chemotherapy for treatment of patients with advanced, refractory malignancies. Cancer Treat Rep 66:259–265

Herman TS, Henle KJ, Nagle WA, Moss AJ, Monson TP (1984a) Effect of step down heating on the cytotoxicity of adriamycin, bleomycin, and cis-diamminedichloroplatinum. Cancer Res 44:1823–1826

Herman TS, Henle KJ, Nagle WA, Moss AJ, Monson TP (1984b) Exposure to pretreatment hypothermia as a determinant of heat killing. Radiat Res 98:345–353

Hill CR (ed) (1982) Ultrasound, microwave, and radiofrequency radiations: the basis for their potential in cancer therapy. Br J Cancer 45 [Suppl 5]:1–257

Hiramoto R, Ghanta VK, Lilly MB (1984) Reduction of tumor burden in a murine osteosarcoma following hyperthermia combined with cyclophosphamide. Cancer Res 44:1405–1408

Hofer KG, Mivechi NF (1980) Mammalian cell sensitivity to hyperthermia as a function of extracellular and intracellular pH. JNCI 65:621–625

Hofer KG, Choppin DA, Hofer MG (1976) Effect of hyperthermia on the radiosensitivity of normal and malignant cells in mice. Cancer 38:379–387

Holohan EV, Highfield DP, Holahan PK, Dewey WC (1984) Hyperthermic killing and hyperthermic radiosensitization in

Chinese hamster ovary cells: effects of pH and thermal tolerance. Radiat Res 97:108–131

Honess DJ (1983) Animal models in the evaluation of therapeutic gain of thermochemotherapy. In: Spitzky KH (ed) Proceedings of the 13th international congress of chemotherapy, Vienna, August 1983, p 273

Honess DJ, Bleehen NM (1982) Sensitivity of normal mouse marrow and RIF-1 tumor to hyperthermia combined with cyclophosphamide or BCNU: a lack of therapeutic gain. Br J Cancer 46:236–248

Honess DJ, Bleehen NM (1985 a) Potentiation of melphalan by systemic hyperthermia in mice: therapeutic gain for mouse lung microtumours. Int J Hyperthermia 1:57–68

Honess DJ, Bleehen NM (1985 b) Thermochemotherapy with cis-platinum, CCNU, BCNU, chlorambucil and melphalan on murine marrow and two tumors: therapeutic gain for melphalan only. Br J Radiol 58:63–72

Honess DJ, Donaldson J, Workman P, Bleehen NM (1985) The effect of systemic hyperthermia on melphalan pharmacokinetics in mice. Br J Cancer 51:77–84

Hornback NB (ed) (1984) Hyperthermia and cancer: human clinical trial experience, vol 2. CRC Press, Boca Raton

Honda N, Oda S, Noguchi T, Hayano Y, Iwasaka H, Taniguchi K (1988) Reversibility of effect of systemic hyperthermia at 43 °C. Sugahara T, Saito M (eds) Hyperthermic oncology. Taylor and Francis, London, vol I, p. 310–311

Houdas Y, Ring EFJ (1982) Human body temperature: it measurement and regulation. Plenum, New York, pp 1–238

Hugander A, Robins HI, Martin PA, Schmitt C (1987) Temperature distribution during radiant heat whole body hyperthermia: experimental studies in the dog. Int J Hyperthermia 3:199–208

Ibuchi Y, Tanaka R, Yamada N, Hondo H (1988) Selective heat sensitivity of glioma cell ABS P 2-C-2. Proceedings of the 5th international symposium on hyperthermic oncology

Ishida A, Mizuno S (1982) Effects of hyperthermia and ethanol on the cytotoxicity of bleomycin, adriamycin, cis-diamminedichloroplatinum (II) and macromycin toward HeLa cells. Gann 73:129–131

Izumi A, Shigemasa K, Maeta M (1983) Effects of in vitro hyperthermia on murine and human lymphocytes. Cancer 51:2061–2065

Jampel HD, Duff GW, Gershon RK, Atkins E, Durum SK (1983) Fever and immunoregulation. 3. Hyperthermia augments the primary in vitro humoral immune response. J Exp Med 157:1229–1238

Janoff KA, Moseson D, Nohigren J, Davenport C, Richards C, Fletcher WS (1982) The treatment of stage I melanoma of the extremities with regional hyperthermia isolation perfusion. Ann Surg 196:316–323

Johnson HJ (1940) The action of short radio waves on tissues. III. A comparison of the thermal sensitivities of transplantable tumors in vivo and in vitro. Am J Cancer 38:533–550

Johnson HA, Pavalec M (1973) Thermal enhancement of thio-TEPA cytotoxicity. JNCI 50:903–908

Johnson RE, Ruhl U (1976) Treatment of chronic lymphocytic leukemia with emphasis on total body irradiation. Int J Radiat Oncol Biol Phys 1:387–397

Johnston RL, Rama Rao G, Tompkins WAF, Cain CA (1986) Effects of in vivo ultrasound hyperthermia on natural killer cell cytotoxicity in the hamster. Bioelectromagnetics 7:283–293

Joiner MC, Steel GG, Stephens TC (1982) Response of two mouse tumors to hyperthermia with CCNU or melphalan. Br J Cancer 45:17–27

Joshi DS, Barendsen GW (1984) Hyperthermic modification of drug effectiveness for reproductive death of cultured mammalian cells. Indian J Exp Biol 22:248–250

Jonsson GG, Robins HI, Rankin PW, Blank JL, Jacobson FL, Jacobson MK (1987) Effect of whole body hyperthermia on adenine and pyridine nucleotide pools in human periheral lymphocytes. Int Clin Hyperthermia Soc annual meeting, June 14–17, 1987, Sweden

Jorritsma JBM, Konings AWT (1984) The occurence of DNA strand breaks after hyperthermic treatments of mammalian cells with and without radiation. Radiat Res 98:198–208

Jorritsma JBM, Kampinga HH, Scaf AHJ, Konings AWT (1985) Strand break repair, DNA polymerase activity and heat radiosensitization in thermotolerant cells. Int J Hyperthermia 1:131–145

Kal HB, Hatfield M, Hahn GM (1975) Cell cycle progression of murine sarcoma cells after x-irradiation or heat shock. Radiology 117:215–217

Kalland T, Dahlquist I (1983) Effects of in vitro hyperthermia on human natural killer cells. Cancer Res 43:1842–1846

Kamura T, Aoki K, Nishikawa K, Baba T (1979) Antitumor effect of thermodifferential chemotherapy with carboquone on Ehrlich carcinoma. Gann 70:783–790

Kapp D (1982) Discussion: hyperthermia and drugs. NCI Monogr 61:322

Kapp D, Lord PF (1983) Thermal tolerance to WBH. Int J Radiat Oncol Biol Phys 9:917–921

Karnovsky MJ (1967) The ultrastructural basis of capillary permeability studied with peroxidase as a tracer. J Cell Biol 35:213–236

Karre K, Klein GO, Kiessling R, Klein G, Roder JC (1980) Low natural in vivo resistance to syngeneic leukemias in natural killer deficient mice. Nature 284:624–626

Kase KR, Hahn GM (1976) Comparison of some response to hyperthermia by normal human diploid cells and neoplastic cells from the same origin. Eur J Cancer 12:481–491

Keele CA, Neil E (1971) Samson Wright's applied physiology, 12th edn. Oxford University Press, New York, p 204, 336

Kim JH, Kim SH, Hahn EW (1974) Thermal enhancement of the radiosensitivity using cultured normal and neoplastic cells. AJR 121:860–864

Kim H, Kim JH, Hahn EW (1975 a) The radiosensitization of hypoxic tumor cells by hyperthermia. Radiology 114:727–728

Kim SH, Kim JH, Hahn EW (1975 b) Enhanced killing of hypoxic tumor cells by hyperthermia. Br J Radiol 48:872–874

Kim JH, Kim SH, Hahn EW (1978) 5-Thio-D-glucose selectivity potentiates hyperthermic killing of hypoxic tumor cells. Science 200:206–207

Kim SH, Kim JH, Hahn EW (1978) Selective potentiation of hyperthermic killing of hypoxic cells by 5-thio-D-glucose. Cancer Res 38:2935–2938

Kim JH, Hahn EW (1979) Clinical and biological studies of localized hyperthermia. Cancer Res 39:2258–2262

Kim JH, Hahn EW, Ahmed S (1982) Combined hyperthermia and radiation therapy for malignant melanoma. Cancer 50:478–482

Kim JH, Kim SH, Alfieri AA, Young CW (1984 a) Quercetin, an inhibitor of lactate transport and a hyperthermic sensitizer of HeLa cells. Cancer Res 44:102–106

Kim JH, Kim SH, Alfieri AA, Young CW, Silvestrini B (1984 b) Lonidamine: a hyperthermic sensitizer of HeLa cells in culture and of the meth-A tumor in vivo. Oncology 41:30–35

Kim SH, Kim JH, Hahn EW, Ensign NA (1980) Selective killing of glucose and oxygen-deprived HeLa cells by hyperthermia. Cancer Res 40:3459–3462

Kim YD, Lees DE, Lake CR, Whang-Peng J, Schutte W, Smith R, Bull J (1979a) Hyperthermia potentiates doxorubicin-related cardiotoxic effects. J Am Med Assoc 241:1816–1817

Kim YD, Raymond Lake C, Lees DE, Schuette WH, Bull JM, Weise V, Kopin IJ (1979b) Hemodynamic and plasma catecholamine responses to hyperthermia cancer therapy in humans. Am J Physiol 237:H570

Klein ME, Frayer K, Bachur NR (1977) Hyperthermic enhancement of chemotherapeutic agents in L1210 leukemia. Blood 50 [Suppl]:223

Klostergaard J, Barta M, Tomasovic SP (1989) Hyperthermic modulation of tumor necrosis factor-dependent monocyte/macrophage tumor cytotoxicity in vitro. J Biol Response Mod 8:262–277

Kluger MJ (1980) Historical aspects of fever and its role in disease. In: Cox B, Lomay P, Milton AS, Schönbaum E (eds) Thermoregulatory mechanisms and their therapeutic implications. 4th international symposium on pharmacology of thermoregulation. Karger, Basel, pp 65–70

Knochel JP (1977) The pathophysiology and clinical characteristics of severe hypophosphatemia. Arch Intern Med 137:203

Koga S, Akio I, Maeta M, Shimazu N, Osaki Y, Kanayoma H (1983) The effects of total body hyperthermia combined with anticancer drugs on immunity in advanced cancer patients. Cancer 52:1173–1177

Koga S, Hamazoe R, Maeta M, Shimizu N, Kanayama H, Osaki Y (1984) Treatment of implanted peritoneal cancer in rats by continuous hyperthermic peritoneal perfusion in combination with an anticancer drug. Cancer Res 44:1840–1842

Koga S, Maeta M, Shimizu N, Osaki Y, Hamazoe R, Masayuki O, Karino T, Yamane T (1985) Clinical effects of total-body hyperthermia combined with anticancer chemotherapy for far-advanced gastrointestinal cancer. Cancer 55:1641–1647

Kohn KW (1977) Interstrand cross-linking of DNA by 1,3 bis(2-chloroethyl)1-nitrosourea and other 1-(2-haloethyl)-1-nitrosoureas. Cancer Res 37:1450–1454

Kremkau FW, Kaufman JS, Walker MM, Burch PG, Spurr CL (1976) Ultrasonic enhancement of nitrogen mustard cytotoxicity in mouse leukemia. Cancer 37:1643–1647

Kubota Y, Nishimura R, Takai S, Umeda M (1979) Effect of hyperthermia on DNA single strand breaks by bleomycin in HeLa cells. Gann 70:681–685

Kwok L, Lin P, Hefter K, Wallach DFH (1978) Impairment of Na^+-dependent amino acid transport in a cultured human T-cell line by hyperthermia and irradiation. Cancer Res 38:83–87

Lange I, Zanker KS, Siewert JR, Blumel G, Eisler K, Kolb E (1984) The effect of whole body hyperthermia on 5-fluorouracil pharmacokinetics in vivo and clonogenicity of mammalian colon cancer cells. Anticancer Res 4:27–32

Langer M, Weidenmaier W, Rottinger EM (1982) Increased cytotoxicity of misonidazole by pH reduction and 41 °C hyperthermia in Chinese hamster cells. Strahlentherapie 158:688–691

Larkin JM (1979) A clinical investigation of total body hyperthermia as a cancer therapy. Cancer Res 39:2252–2254

Larkin J, Edwards WS, Smith DE, Clark PJ (1977) Systemic thermotherapy: description of a method and physiologic tolerance in clinical subjects. Cancer 40:3155–3159

Law HT, Pettigrew RT (1980) Heat transfer in whole body hyperthermia. Ann NY Acad Sci 335:298

Law MP, Ahier RG, Field SB (1977) The response of mouse skin to combined hyperthermia and x-rays. Int J Radiat Biol 32:153–163

Lazo JS, Braun D, Meandzija B, Kennedy KA, Pham ET, Smaldone LF (1985) Lidocaine potentiation of bleomycin A2 cytotoxicity and DNA strand breakage in L1210 and human A-253 cells. Cancer Res 45:2103–2109

Lees DE, Kim YD, Dubois M, Bull JM, Smith R, Schuette WH, MacNamara TG (1982) Internal organ hypoxia during hyperthermia cancer therapy in humans. NCI Monogr 61:339–401

Lehman CM, Stewart JR (1983) In vivo cytotoxicity of misonidazole and hyperthermia in a transplanted mouse mammary tumor. Radiat Res 96:628–634

Lele PP, Parker KJ (1982) Temperature distributions in tissues during local hyperthermia by stationary or steered beams of unfocused and focused ultrasound. Br J Cancer 45 [Suppl]:108–121

LeVeen HH, Wapnick S, Piccone V, Falk G, Ahmed N (1976) Tumor eradication by radiofrequency therapy. J Am Med Assoc 235:2198–2200

Levin W, Blair RM (1978) Clinical experience with combined whole-body hyperthermia and radiation. In: Streffer S, van Beuningen D, Dietzel F et al. (eds) Cancer therapy by hyperthermia and radiation. Urban and Schwarzenberg, Baltimore, pp 322–325

Levin W, Blair RM (1982) Pettigrew technique of inducing whole body hyperthermia. In: Cancer therapy by hyperthermia, drugs and radiation. NCI Monogr 61:377

Li DJ, Hahn GM (1983) Effects of ethanol and whole body hyperthermia on survival of mice. Radiat Res 94:564

Li DJ, Hahn GM (1984) Response of RIF tumors to heat and drugs: dependence on tumor size. Cancer Treat Rep 68:1149–1151

Li GC (1984) Thermal biology and physiology in clinical hyperthermia: current status and future needs. Cancer Res [Suppl] 44:4886 s–4893 s

Li GC, Hahn GM (1978) Ethanol induces tolerance to heat and to adriamycin. Nature 274:699–701

Li GC, Kal HB (1977) Effect of hyperthermia on the radiation response of two mammalian cell lines. Eur J Cancer 13:65–69

Lilly JK, Boland JP, Zekan S (1980) Urinary bladder temperature monitoring: A new index of body core temperature. Crit Care Med 8:742–744

Lin PS, Wallach DFH, Tsai S (1973) Temperature-induced variations in the surface topology of cultured lymphocytes are revealed by scanning electron microscopy. Prog Natl Acad Sci USA 70:2492–2496

Lin PS, Cariani PA, Jones M, Kahn PC (1983a) Work in progress: the effect of heat on bleomycin cytotoxicity in vitro and on the accumulation of cobleomycin in heat-treated rat tumors. Radiology 146:213–217

Lin PS, Hefter K, Jones M (1983b) Hyperthermia and bleomycin schedules on V79 Chinese hamster cell cytotoxicity in vitro. Cancer Res 43:4557–4561

Loehrer PJ, Einhorn LH (1984) Drugs five years later: cisplatin. Ann Intern Med 100:704–713

Longo FW, Tomaschevsky P, Rivin BD, Tannenbaum M (1983) Interaction of ultrasonic hyperthermia with two alkylating agents in a murine bladder tumor. Cancer Res 43:3231–3235

Lord PF, Kapp DS, Morrow D (1981) Increased skeletal metastases of spontaneous canine osteosarcoma after fractionated systemic hyperthermia and local x-irradiation. Cancer Res 41:4331–4334

Lorenz M, Habs M, Schmahl D (1983) Effect of moderate local hyperthermia combined with chemotherapy by administration of cyclophosphamide or nitroso 1,3 bis(2-chloroethyl)urea (BCNU) on Yoshida sarcoma implanted in the descending colon of rats. Langenbecks Arch Chir 359: 205–213

Loshek DD, Greenlaw RH, Doyle LA (1981) Whole body

hyperthermia using a water circulator. Strahlentherapie 157:620–621

Loven D, Lurie H, Hazan G (1986) Enhanced effect of systemic cyclophosphamide by local tumor hyperthermia in mice. Cancer Treat Rep 70:509–512

Ludlum DB (1977) Alkylating agents and nitrosoureas. In: Becker SF (ed) Cancer: a comprehensive treatise, vol 5. Plenum, New York, pp 285–307

Luk KH, Purser PR, Castro JR, Meyler TS, Phillips TL (1981) Clinical experiences with local microwave hyperthermia. Int J Radiat Oncol Biol Phys 7:615–620

Lunec J, Hesselwood IP, Parker R, Leaper S (1981) Hyperthermic enhancement of radiation cell killing in HeLa S3 cells and its effect on the production and repair of DNA strand breaks. Radiat Res 85:116–125

Macy DW, Gasper PW (1988) Effect of whole body hyperthermia on cats infected with feline leukemia virus. Veterinary Cancer Society 8th annual conference

Macy DW, Macy CA, Scott RJ, Gillette EL, Speer JF (1985) Physiological studies of whole-body hyperthermia of dogs. Cancer Res 45:2769–2773

Maeta M, Koga S, Wada J, Yokoyama M, Kato N, Kawahara H, Sakai T, Hino M, Ono T, Yuasa K (1987) Clinical evaluation of total-body hyperthermia combined with anticancer chemotherapy for far-advanced miscellaneous cancer in Japan. Cancer 59:1101–1106

Mahaley MS Jr, Woodhall B (1961) Effect of temperature upon the in vitro action of anticancer agents on VX2 carcinoma. J Neurosurg 18:269–272

Magin RL, Niesman MR (1984) Temperature-dependent permeability of large unilamellar liposomes. Chem Phys Lipids 34:245–256

Magin RL, Sikic BI, Cytsyk RL (1979) Enhancement of bleomycin activity against Lewis lung tumors in mice by local hyperthermia. Cancer Res 39:3792–3795

Magin RL, Cytsyk RL, Litterst CL (1980) Distribution of adriamycin in mice under conditions of local hyperthermia which improve systemic drug therapy. Cancer Treat Rep 64:203–210

Malangoni MA, Grosfeld JL, Cakmak O, Ballantine TVN (1978) The effect of hyperthermia on survival in transplanted lymphosarcoma. J Pediatr Surg 13:740–745

Mann BD, Storm FK, Morton DL (1983) Predictability of response to clinical thermochemotherapy by the clonogenic assay. Cancer 52:1389–1394

Manning MR, Cetas TC, Miller RC, Oleson JR, Connor WG, Gerner EW (1982) Clinical hyperthermia: results of a Phase I trial employing hyperthermia alone or in combination with external beam or interstitial radiotherapy. Cancer 49:205–216

Marchal C, Anghileri LJ, Escanye MC, Robert J (1986) Hyperthermia and cytotoxic drugs. Possible use of lanthanum as a potentiator of hyperthermia. Int J Hyperthermia 2:83–92

Marmor JB (1979) Interactions of hyperthermia and chemotherapy in animals. Cancer Res 39:2269–2276

Marmor JB (1983) Cancer therapy by ultrasound. Adv Radiat Biol 10:105–133

Marmor JB, Hahn GM (1980) Combined radiation and hyperthermia in superficial human tumors. Cancer 46:1986–1991

Marmor JB, Hahn N, Hahn GM (1977) Tumor cure and cell survival after localized radiofrequency heating. Cancer Res 37:879–883

Marmor JB, Kozak D, Hahn GM (1979a) Effects of systemically administered bleomycin or adriamycin with local hyperthermia on primary tumor and lung metastases. Cancer Treat Rep 63:1311–1325

Marmor JB, Pounds D, Postic TB, Hahn GM (1979b) Treatment of superficial human neoplasms by local hyperthermia induced ultrasound. Cancer 43:188–197

Martin LS, McDougal JS, Lorkoski SL (1985) Disinfection and inactivation of the human T-lymphotropic virus type III, lymphadenopathy-associated virus. J Infect Dis 152:400–403

Martin PA, Robins HI, Dennis WH (1987) Monitoring body site temperature during systemic hyperthermia. Crit Care Med 15:163–164

Maxwell GM, Castillo CA, Crumpton CW, Rowe GG (1959) Hyperthermia: systemic and coronary circulatory changes in the intact dog. Am Heart J 58:854–862

McDougal JS, Martin LS, Cart SP et al. (1985) Thermal inactivation of the acquired immunodeficiency syndrome virus human T-lymphotropic virus III, lymphadenopathy-associated virus, with special reference to antihemophilic factor. J Clin Invest 76:875–876

McTaggart HS, Laing AH, Imlah P, Head KW, Brownlie SE (1979) The genetics of hereditary lymphosarcoma of pigs. Vet Rec 105:39

Mella O (1985) Combined hyperthermia and cis-diamminedichloroplatinum in BDIX rats with transplanted BT4A tumors. Int J Hyperthermia 1:171–183

Merritt JA, Meltzer DM, Ball LA, Borden EC (1985) 2-5A synthetase activity in patients with metastatic carcinoma and its response to interferon treatment. In: Williams B, Silverman R (eds) The 2-5A system, molecular aspects. Liss, New York, pp 423–430

Meyer JL (1984a) The clinical efficacy of localized hyperthermia. Cancer Res 44:4745a–4751s

Meyer JL (1984b) Hyperthermia as an anticancer modality – a historical perspective. Front Radiat Ther Oncol 18:1–22

Meyer RE, Page RL, Thrall DE, Dewhirst MW, Vose DL (1986) Determination of continuous atracurium infusion rate in dogs undergoing whole-body hyperthermia. Cancer Res 46:5599–5601

Meyn RE, Corry PM, Fletcher SE, Demetriades M (1980) Thermal enhancement of DNA damage in mammalian cells treated with cis-diamminedichloroplatinum (II). Cancer Res 40:1136–1139

Miller RC, Leith JT, Veomett RC, Gerner EW (1976) Potentiation of radiation myelitis in rats by hyperthermia. Br J Radiol 49:895–896

Milligan AJ (1984) Whole-body hyperthermia induction techniques. Cancer Res [Suppl] 44:4869s–4872s

Mills MD, Meyn RE (1981) Effects of hyperthermia on repair of radiation-induced DNA strand breaks. Radiat Res 87:314–328

Mills MS, Meyn RE (1983) Hyperthermic potentiation of unrejoined DNA strand breaks following irradiation. Radiat Res 95:327–338

Milnor WR, Bergel DH, Bargainer JD (1966) Hydraulic Power associated with pulmonary blood flow and its relation to heart rate. Circulation Res 19(3):467–480

Mimnaugh EG, Waring RW, Sikic BI, Magin RL, Drew R, Litterst CL, Gram TE, Guarino AM (1978) Effect of whole-body hyperthermia on the disposition and metabolism of adriamycin in rabbits. Cancer Res 38:1420–1425

Mini E, Dombrowski J, Moroson BA, Bertino JR (1986) Cytotoxic effects of hyperthermia, 5-fluorouracil and their combination on a human leukemia T-lymphoblast cell line, CCRF-CEM. Eur J Cancer Clin Oncol 22:927–934

Minna JD, Pass H, Glatstein E, Ihde DC (1989) Cancer of the lung. In: DeVita Jr VT, Hellman S, Rosenberg SA (eds) Cancer, principles and practice of oncology, 3rd edn. Lippincott, Philadelphia, pp 591–705

Mivechi NF, Hofer KG (1983) Evidence for separtate modes of

action in thermal radiosensitization and direct thermal cell death. Cancer 51:38–43

Mivechi NF, Li GC (1987) Lack of effect of thermotolerance on radiation response and thermal radiosensitization of murine bone marrow progenitors. Cancer Res 47:1538–1541

Miyakoshi J, Heki S, Furukawa M, Kano E (1982) Recovery kinetics from the damage by step-up and step-down heatings in combination with radiation in Chinese hamster cells. J Radiat Res 23:187–197

Mizel SB (1989) The interleukins. FASEB J 3:2379

Mizuno S (1981) Ethanol-induced sensitization to bleomycin cytotoxicity and the inhibition of recovery from potentially lethal damage. Cancer Res 41:4111–4114

Mizuno S, Ishida A (1981) Potentiation of bleomycin cytotoxicity toward cultured mouse cells by hyperthermia and ethanol. Gann 72:395–402

Mizuno S, Ishida A (1982) Selective enhancement of the cytotoxicity of the bleomycin derivative, peplomycin by local anesthetics alone and combined with hyperthermia. Cancer Res 42:4726–4729

Mizuno S, Amagai M, Ishida A (1980) Synergistic cell killing by antitumor agents and hyperthermia in cultured cells. Gann 71:471–478

Mole RH (1953) Whole body irradiation – radiobiology or medicine? Br J Radiol 26:234–240

Mondovi B, Santoro AS, Strom R, Faiola R, Rossi-Fanelli A (1972) Increased immunogenicity of Ehrlich ascites cells after heat treatment. Cancer 30:885–888

Moore M (1978) Antigens of experimentally induced neoplasms: a conspectus. In: Castro JE (ed) Immunol aspects of cancer. MTP Press, Lancaster, pp 15–50

Morgan JE, Bleehan NM (1981 a) Response of EMT6 multicellular tumor spheroids to hyperthermia. Br J Cancer 43:384–391

Morgan JE, Bleehan NM (1981 b) Interactions between misonidazole and hyperthermia in EMT6 spheroids. Br J Cancer 44:810–818

Morgan JE, Honess D, Bleehan N (1979) The interaction of thermal tolerance with drug cytotoxicity in vitro. Br J Cancer 39:422–428

Moricca G, Cavaliere R, Caputo A (1977) Hyperthermic treatment of tumors: experimental and clinical observations. In: Rentchnick P et al. (eds) Recent results in cancer research, vol 59. Springer, Berlin Heidelberg New York, pp 112–152

Morris CC, Myers R, Field SB (1977) Response of the rat tail to hyperthermia. Br J Radiol 50:576–580

Muckle DS, Dickson JA (1973) Hyperthermia (42 °C) as an adjuvant to radiotherapy and chemotherapy in the treatment of the allogeneic VX2 carcinoma in the rabbit. Br J Cancer 27:307–315

Mullbacher A (1984) Hyperthermia and the generation and activity of murine influenza – immune cytotoxic T cells in vitro. J Virol 52:928–931

Murray D, Milas L, Meyn RE (1984) DNA damage produced by combined hyperglycemia and hyperthermia in two mouse fibrosarcoma tumors in vivo. Int J Radiat Oncol Biol Phys 10:1679–1682

Myers R, Field SB (1977) The response of rat tails to combined heat and x-rays. Br J Radiol 50:581–586

Nakajima K, Hisazumi H (1983) An experimental study of enhanced cell killing by hyperthermia and bleomycin. Urol Res 11:43–46

Nauts HC, Fowler GA, Bogatko FH (1953) A review of the influence of bacterial infections and bacterial products (Coley's toxins) on malignant tumors in men. Acta Med Scand [Suppl] 276:1–103

Nelson TE, Flewellen EH (1983) The malignant hyperthermia syndrome. N Engl J Med 309:416

Neumann H, Fabricius HA, Engelhardt R (1982) Moderate whole-body hyperthermia in combination with chemotherapy in the treatment of small cell carcinoma of the lung: a pilot study. NCI Monogr 61:427

Neumann HA, Fiebig HH, Lohr GW, Engelhardt R (1985) Effects of cytostatic drugs and 40.5 °C hyperthermia on human bone marrow progenitors (CFU-C) and human clonogenic tumor cells implanted into mice. JNCI 75:1059–1066

Neumann HA, Hermann DJB, Engelhardt R (1988) Changes of plasma acetate levels in whole body hyperthermia. In: Issels RD, Wilmanns W (eds) Application of hyperthermia in the treatment of cancer. Springer, Berlin Heidelberg New York, pp 27–31 (Recent results in cancer research, vol 107)

Neville AJ, Sauder DN (1988) Whole body hyperthermia (41 °–42 °C) induces interleukin-1 in vivo. Lymphokine Res 7:201–206

Neville AJ, Robins HI, Martin PA, Gilchrist KW, Dennis WH, Steeves RA (1984) Effect of whole body hyperthermia and BCNU on the development of radiation myelitis in the rat. Int J Radiat Biol 46:417–420

Neville AJ, Robins HI, Longo WL, Konick K, Gilchrist KW (1986) A case report of leptomeningeal involvement of pancreatic carcinoma following whole body hyperthermia and pancreatic irradiation. Cancer J 1:132–134

Nielson OS (1983) Influence of thermotolerance on the interaction between hyperthermia and radiation in L1A2 cells in vitro. Int J Radiat Biol 43:665–673

Nielson OS, Overgaard J (1979) Effect of extracellular pH on thermotolerance and recovery of hyperthermic damage in vitro. Cancer Res 39:2772–2778

Nielson OS, Overgaard J, Kamura T (1983) Influence of thermotolerance on the interaction between hyperthermia and radiation in a solid tumor in vivo. Br J Radiol 56:267–273

Niitsu Y, Watanabe N, Umeno H, Sone H, Neda H, Yamauchi N, Maeda M, Urushizaki I (1988) Synergistic effects of recombinant human tumor necrosis factor and hyperthermia on in vitro cytotoxicity and artificial metastasis. Cancer Res 48:654–657

Noodleman FR, Koperski JA, Pounds D, Farber EM, Orenberg EK (1984) Thermal dosimetry evaluations of normal human skin and psoriatic plaques. Proc Rad Res Soc ABS DC-9, p 22

Nurmi T, Uhari M, Kouvalainen K (1982) Temperature and natural killer cell activity. Lancet 1:516–517

Nussbaum GH (ed) (1982) Physical aspects of hyperthermia. American Institute of Physics, New York, Medical Physics Monograph 8

Oda M, Koga S, Maeta M (1985) Effects of total-body hyperthermia on metastases from experimental mouse tumors. Cancer Res 45:1532–1535

O'Donnell JF, Mockoy WS, Makuch RW, Bull JM (1979) Increased in vitro toxicity to mouse bone marrow with 1,3 bis(2-chloroethyl)1-nitrosourea and hyperethermia. Cancer Res 39:2547–2549

Ohnoshi T, Ohnuma T, Beranek JT, Holland JF (1985) Combined cytotoxicity effect of hyperthermia and anthracycline antibiotics on human tumor cells. JNCI 74:275–281

Oleson JR (1982) Hyperthermia by magnetic induction: I. Physical characteristics of the technique. Int J Radiat Oncol Biol Phys 8:1747–1756

Oleson JR, Dewhirst MW (1983) Hyperthermia: an overview of current progress and problems. Curr Probl Cancer 8:1–62

Oleson JR, Heusinkveld RS, Manning MR (1983) Hyperthermia by magnetic induction: II. Clinical experience with concentric electrodes. Int J Radiat Oncol Biol Phys 9:549–556

Oleson JR, Manning MR, Sim DA, Heusinkveld RS, Aristizabal SA, Cetas TC, Hevezi JM, Connor WG (1984a) A review of the University of Arizona human clinical hyperthermia experience. Front Radiat Ther Oncol 18:136–143

Oleson J, Sim D, Manning M (1984b) Analysis of prognostic variables in hyperthermia treatment of 161 patients. Int J Radiat Oncol Biol Phys 10:2231–2240

Ono S, Strebel F, Baba H, Stephens LC, Khokhar AR, Siddik ZH, Bull JMC (1990) Effect of whole body hyperthermia combined with carboplatin on tumor and normal tissue in rats. Proc NAHG/38th Radiat Res Soc

Onsrud M (1983) Effects of hyperthermia on human natural killer cells. Acta Pathol Microbiol Immunol Scand [C]91:1–8

Orth PE, Swidler HJ, Zarakov MS (1977) Survival of pleomorphic sarcoma-37 transplanted in virgin female DBA/2J mice: hyperthermia and hyperglycemia, alone or in combination with drugs. J Pharm Sci 66:437–438

Ostrow S, Van Echo D, Whitacre M, Aisner J, Simon R, Wiernik PH (1981) Physiologic response and toxicity in patients undergoing whole-body hyperthermia for the treatment of cancer. Cancer Treat Rep 65:323–325

Overgaard J (1976) Combined adriamycin and hyperthermia treatment of a murine mammary carcinoma in vivo. Cancer Res 36:3077–3081

Overgaard J (1980) Simultaneous and sequential hyperthermia and radiation treatment of an experimental tumor and its surrounding normal tissue in vivo. Int J Radiat Oncol Biol Phys 6:1507–1517

Overgaard J (1981a) Fractionated radiation and hyperthermia. Experimental and clinical studies. Cancer 48:1116–1123

Overgaard J (1981b) Effect of hyperthermia on the hypoxic fraction of an experimental mammary carcinoma in vivo. Br J Radiol 54:245–249

Overgaard J (1984) Formula to estimate the thermal enhancement of ratio of a single simultaneous hyperthermia and radiation treatment. Acta Radiol Oncol 23:135–139

Overgaard J, Nielson OS (1983) The importance of thermotolerance for the clinical treatment with hyperthermia. Radiat Oncol 1:167–178

Overgaard K, Overgaard J (1972) Investigations on the possibility of a thermic tumor therapy II. Eur J Cancer 8:573–575

Page RL, Macy DW, Thrall DE, Dewhirst MW, Allen SL, Heidner GL, Sim DA, McGee ML, Gillette EL (1988) Unexpected toxicity associated with use of body surface area for dosing melphalan in the dog. Cancer Res 48:288–290

Page RL, McEntee MC, Heidner GL, Riviere JE, Thrall DE (1989) Phase I evaluation of carboplatin at 37° and 42°C in tumor-bearing dogs. Proc Radiat Res Soc NAHG Abstract Bd-9

Palzer RJ, Heidelberger C (1973a) Studies on the quantitative biology of hyperthermic cell killing of HeLa cells. Cancer Res 33:415–421

Palzer RJ, Heidelberger C (1973b) Influence of drugs and synchrony on the hyperthermic killing of HeLa cells. Cancer Res 33:422–427

Parks LC, Smith GV (1983) Systemic hyperthermia by extracorporeal induction: techniques and results. In: Storm FK (ed) Hyperthermia in cancer therapy. Hall, Boston, pp 407–446

Parks LC, Turner MD, Minaberry D, Grogan J, Douglas M, Neely WA, Hardy JD (1978) Anticancer hyperthermia. Metabolic, physiologic and immunologic responses of man. Fed Proc Am Soc Exp Biol 37:930

Parks LC, Minaberry D, Smith DP, Neeley WA (1979) Treatment of far-advanced bronchogenic carcinoma by extracorporeally induced systemic hyperthermia. J Thorac Cardiovasc Surg 78:883–892

Patton JF, Doolittle WH (1972) Core rewarming by peritoneal dialysis following induced hypothermia in the dog. J Appl Physiol 33:800–804

Pettigrew RT, Ludgate C (1977) Whole body hyperthermia, a systemic treatment for disseminated cancer. In: Rentchnick et al. (eds) Recent results in cancer research, vol 59. Springer, Berlin Heidelberg New York, pp 153–170

Pettigrew RT, Galt JM, Ludgate CM, Horn DB, Smith AN (1974a) Circulatory and biochemical effects of whole body hyperthermia. Br J Surg 61:727–730

Pettigrew RT, Galt JM, Ludgate CM, Smith AN (1974b) Clinical effects of whole body hyperthermia in advanced malignancy. Br Med J 61:679–682

Philip R, Epstein LB (1986) Tumor necrosis factor as immunomodulator and mediator of monocyte cytotoxicity induced by itself, gamma-interferon, and interleukin-1. Nature 323:86–89

Pickering BG, Bristow GK, Craig DB (1977) Core rewarming by peritoneal irrigation in accidental hypothermia with cardiac arrest. Anesth Analg 56:574–577

Pilepich MV, Myerson RJ, Emaml BN, Perez CA, Leybovich L, Von Gerichien D (1987) Regional hyperthermia: a feasibility analysis. Int J Hyperthermia 3:347–351

Poli G, Kinter A, Justement JS, Kehrl JH, Bressler P, Stanley S, Fauci AS (1990) Tumor necrosis factor-alpha functions in an autocrine manner in the induction of HIV expression. Proc Natl Acad Sci USA 87:782–785

Pomp H (1978) Clinical application of hyperthermia in gynecological malignant tumors. In: Streffer C, Van Beuningen D, Dietzel F et al. (eds) Cancer therapy by hyperthermia and radiation. Urban and Schwarzenberg, Baltimore, p 326

Pozos RS, Wittmers LE (eds) (1983) The nature and treatment of hypothermia. University of Minnesota Press, Minneapolis, pp 1–277

Priesching A (1976) Hyperthermie in der Krebsbehandlung? In: Schmähl D (ed) Prophylaxe und Therapie von Behandlungsfolgen bei Karzinomen der Frau; 2. Oberaudorfer Gespräch, Oct 1975. Thieme, Stuttgart, pp 56–64

Price GS, Page RL, Riviere JE, Cline JM, Thrall DE (1989) Pharmacokinetics and toxicity of intravenous lonidamine and whole body hyperthermia in normal dogs. Radiat Res, NAHG, Ci-22, p 69

Primm MV, Baldwin RW (1978) Immunology and immunotherapy of experimental and clinical metastases. In: Baldwin RW (ed) Secondary spread of cancer. Academic, London, pp 163–209

Prionas SD, Taylor MA, Fajardo LF, Kelly NI, Nelsen TS, Hahn GM (1985) Thermal sensitivity to single and double heat treatments in normal canine liver. Cancer Res 45:4791–4797

Pritsos CA, Sartorelli AC (1986) Generation of reactive oxygen radicals through bioactivation of mitomycin antibiotics. Cancer Res 46:3528–3532

Raaphorst GP, Azzam EL (1983) Thermal radiosensitization in Chinese hamster (V79) and mouse C3H 10T1/2 cells. The thermotolerance effect. Br J Cancer 48:45–54

Raaphorst GP, Romano SL, Mitchell JB, Bedford JS, Dewey WC (1971) Intrinsic differences in heat and/or x-ray sensitivity of seven mammalian cell lines cultured and treated under identical conditions. Cancer Res 39:396–401

Raaphorst GP, Szekely J, Lobeau A, Azzam EI (1983) A comparison of cell killing by heat and/or x-rays in Chinese hamster V79 cells, Friend erythroleukemia mouse cells, and human thymocyte MOLT-4 cells. Radiat Res 94:340–349

Radford IR (1983) Effects of hyperthermia on the repair of x-ray induced DNA double strand breaks in mouse L cells. Int J Radiat Biol Relat Stud Phys Chem Med 43:551–557

Rege VB, Leone LA, Soderberg CH, Coleman GV, Robidoux HJ, Fijman R, Brown J (1983) Hyperthermic adjuvant perfusion chemotherapy for stage I malignant melanoma of the extremity with literature review. Cancer 52:2033–2039

Resnick L, Veren K, Salahuddin SZ, Tonrewau S, Markham PD (1986) Stability and inactivation of HLTV-III/LAV under clinical and laboratory environments. J Am Med Assoc 255:1887–1891

Reuler JB (1978) Hypothermia: pathophysiology, clinical setting and management. Ann Intern Med 89:519–527

Ritter MA, Cleaver JE, Tobias CA (1977) High-LET radiations induce a large proportion of nonrejoining DNA breaks. Nature 266:653–655

Riviere JE, Page RL, Dewhirst MW, Tyczkowska K, Thrall DE (1986) Effect of hyperthermia on cisplatin pharmacokinetics in normal dogs. Int J Hyperthermia 2:351–358

Roberts NJ Jr, Stiegbigel RT (1977) Hyperthermia and human leukocyte functions: effects on response of lymphocytes to mitogen and antigen and bactericidal capacity of monocytes and neutrophils. Infect Immun 18:673–679

Roberts NJ Jr, Lu ST, Michaelson SM (1985) Hyperthermia and human leukocyte functions: DNA, RNA, and total protein synthesis after exposure to $<41°$ or $>42.5°$ hyperthermia. Cancer Res 45:3076–3082

Robins HI (1984) The role of whole body hyperthermia in the treatment of neoplastic disease, its current status and future prospects. Cancer Res 44:4878s–4883s

Robins HI (1988) Whole body hyperthermia: the University of Wisconsin Clinical Cancer Center experience. In: Paliwal BR, Hetzel FR, Dewhirst MW (eds) Physical aspects of hyperthermia, American Association of Physicists, in: Medicine (AAPM) Monograph 16, American Institute of Physics Publication Division, New York, pp 345–355

Robins HI (1989) Hyperthermia as cancer therapy: current status and future prospects. In: McGrath IT (ed) New directions in cancer treatment – UICC. Springer, Berlin Heidelberg New York, pp 85–92

Robins HI, Neville AJ (1986) Biology and methodology of whole body hyperthermia. In: Anghileri LV, Robert J (eds) Hyperthermia in cancer treatment, vol 3. CRC Press, Boca Raton, pp 183–206

Robins HI, Steeves RA, Miller KH, Yatvin MB (1982) The differential sensitivity of murine AKR leukemia and normal bone marrow cells to hyperthermia and lidocaine. Radiat Res 91:321

Robins HI, Dennis WH, Slattery JS, Lange TA, Yatvin MB (1983a) Systemic lidocaine enhancement of hyperthermia-induced tumor regression in transplantable murine models. Cancer Res 43:3187–3191

Robins HI, Grossman J, Davis TE, Dennis WH, AuBuchon JP (1983b) A preclinical trial of a radiant heat device for whole body hyperthermia using a porcine model. Cancer Res 43:2018–2022

Robins HI, Shecterle LM, AuBuchon JP, Paliwal BR, Davis TE, Dennis WH (1983c) Whole body hyperthermia with a microwave regional boost: unexpected toxicity in the pig. Int J Radiat Biol 44:469–473

Robins HI, Steeves RA, Martin PA, Miller K, Clark AW, Dennis WH (1983d) Differential sensitivity of AKR murine leukemia and normal bone marrow cells to hyperthermia. Cancer Res 43:4951–4955

Robins HI, Dennis WH, Martin PA, Sondel PM, Yatvin MB, Steeves RA (1984a) Potentiation of differential hyperthermic sensitivity of AKR leukemia and normal bone marrow cells by lidocaine or thiopental. Cancer 54:2831–2835

Robins HI, Dennis WH, Steeves RA, Sondel PM (1984b) A proposal for the addition of hyperthermia to treatment regimens for acute and chronic leukemia. J Clin Oncol 2:1050–1056

Robins HI, Steeves RA, Shecterle LM, Martin PA, Miller KA, Paliwal B, Neville AJ, Dennis WH (1984c) Whole body hyperthermia (41 °–42 °C): a simple technique for unanesthetized mice. Med Phys 11:833–839

Robins HI, Dennis WH, Neville AJ, Hugander A, Shecterle LM, Martin PA, Gillis WK, Grossman J, Steeves RA, Davis TE (1985a) Whole body hyperthermia clinical trials. Proc IEEE/Engineering Medicine and Biology Society 1:361–364

Robins HI, Denis WH, Neville AJ, Shecterle LM, Martin PA, Grossman J, Davis TE, Neville SR, Gillis WK, Rusy BF (1985b) A nontoxic system for 41.8 °C whole body hyperthermia: results of a Phase I study using a radiant heat device. Cancer Res 45:3937–3944

Robins HI, Hugander A, Steeves R, Dennis WH (1986a) Radiotherapy and hyperthermia for lung cancer. Int J Radiat Oncol Biol Phys 12:147

Robins HI, Longo WL, Hugander A, Bozdeck M, Schwartz B, Steeves RA, Flynn B, Trigg M, Sondel PM (1986b) Whole body hyperthermia combined with total body irradiation and chemotherapy as a preparative regimen for allogenic bone marrow transplantation. Cancer J 1:180–183

Robins HI, Storer B, Longo WL, Sauerssig J, Jendre R, Shecterle LM, Hugander AH, Hawkins MJ, Sielaff KM, Borden EC (1986c) Interferon-alpha (IFN-alpha) and whole body hyperthermia (WBH): a phase I trial. Am Assoc Cancer Res 27:205

Robins HI, Kalin N, Shelton SE, Martin PA, Shecterle LM, Barksdale CN, Neville AJ, Marshall J (1987a) Rise in plasma beta-endorphin, ACTH, and cortisol in cancer patients undergoing whole body hyperthermia. Horm Metab Res 19:441–443

Robins HI, Kalin N, Shelton SE, Shecterle L, Marshal J, Barksdale CN (1987b) Neuroendocrine changes in patients undergoing whole body hyperthermia. Int J Hyperthermia 3:99–105

Robins HI, Longo WL, Lagoni RK, Neville AJ, Riggs C, Schmitt CL, Hugander A, Young C (1988a) A Phase I trial of lonidamine with whole body hyperthermia in advanced cancer. Cancer Res 48:6587–6592

Robins HI, Longo WL, Steeves RA, Lagoni RK, Hugander A, Neville AJ, O'Keefe S, Giese W, Schmitt CL (1988b) A pilot study of whole body hyperthermia and local irradiation for advanced nonsmall cell lung cancer confined to the thorax. Int J Radiat Oncol Biol Phys 15:427–431

Robins HI, Steeves RA, Schmitt CL, Peterson C, Martin PA (1988c) A hyperthermia study of differential sensitivity and thermal tolerance in AKR murine leukemia and normal bone marrow cells. Int J Radiat Oncol Biol Phys 14:979–982

Robins HI, Hugander A, Cohen JD (1989a) Whole body hyperthermia in the treatment of neoplastic disease. In: Steeves RA (ed) Radiologic clinics of North America. Saunders, Philadelphia, pp 603–610

Robins HI, Sielaff KM, Storer B, Hawkins MJ, Borden EC (1989b) A Phase I trial of interferon αLy with whole body hyperthermia in advanced cancer. Cancer Res 49:1609–1615

Robins HI, Longo WL, Steeves RA, Cohen JD, Schmitt CL, Neville AJ, O'Keefe S, Lagoni R, Riggs C (1990a) Adjunctive therapy (whole body hyperthermia versus lonidamine) to total body irradiation for the treatment of favorable B-cell neoplasms: a report of two pilot clinical trials and laboratory investigations. Int J Radiat Oncol Biol Phys 18:909–920

Robins HI, Tutsch K, Cohen J, Schmitt C, Longo W, Javid M, Trump D, Bailey H, Arzoomanian R, Tombes M, Alberti D, Spriggs D (1990b) Phase I clinical trial of carboplatin

(CBDCA) and whole body hyperthermia (WBH). Am Assoc Cancer Res 31:205

Robins HI, Hugander A, Besozzi M, Schmitt CL, Martin PA, Zager LV, Grossman J (1991a) Beta-blockade during whole body hyperthermia: a toxicity study in the dog. Int J Hyperthermia 7:263–270

Robins HI, Jonsson GG, Jacobson EL, Schmitt CL, Jacobson MK, Cohen JD (1991b) Effect of hyperthermia in vitro and in vivo on adenine and pyridine nucleotide pools in human peripheral lymphocytes. Cancer 67:2098–2102

Robinson JE, Wizenberg MJ (1974) Thermal sensitivity and the effect of elevated temperatures on the radiation sensitivity of Chinese hamster cells. Acta Radiol 13:241–248

Robinson JE, Wizenberg MJ, McCready WA (1974) Radiation and hyperthermal response of normal tissue in situ. Radiology 113:195–198

Rofstad EK, Brustad T (1985) Heterogeneity in heat sensitivity and development of thermotolerance of cloned cell lines derived from a single human melanoma xenograft. Int J Hyperthermia 1:85–96

Roizin-Towle L, Hall EJ (1982) Interaction between hyperthermia and cytotoxic agents. NCI Monogr 61:149–151

Rose WC, Veras GH, Laster WR Jr, Schabel FM Jr (1979) Evaluation of whole-body hyperthermia as an adjunct to chemotherapy in murine tumors. Cancer Treat Rep 63:1311–1325

Rossi A, Taricini G, Marchini S, Bonadonna G (1980) Response to secondary treatment after surgical adjuvant CMF for breast cancer. Proc Am Assoc Cancer Res 21:760

Roszkowski W, Szmigielski S, Janiak M, Wrembel JK (1979) Effect of moderate (40 °C) and intensive (43 °C) hyperthermia on spleen, lymph node and thymus-derived murine lymphocytes in vitro. Immunobiology 156:429–440

Roti JL, Winward RT (1978) The effects of hyperthermia on the protein-to-DNA ratio of isolated HeLa cell chromatin. Radiat Res 74:159–169

Rotstein LE, Daly J, Rozsa P (1983) Systemic thermochemotherapy in a rat model. Can J Surg 26:113–116

Rowell LB (1983) Cardiovascular aspects of human thermoregulation. Circ Res 52:367–379

Rozenzweig M, von Hoff DD, Slavik M, Muggia FM (1977) Cis-diamminedichloroplatinum (II), a new anticancer drug. Ann Intern Med 86:803–812

Sapareto SA, Hopwood LE, Dewey WC (1978a) Combined effects of x-irradiation and hyperthermia on CHO cells for various temperatures and orders of application. Radiat Res 73:221–223

Sapareto SA, Hopwood LE, Dewey WC, Raju MR, Gray JW (1978b) Effects of hyperthermia on survival and progression of Chinese hamster ovary cells. Cancer Res 38:393–400

Sapareto SA, Raaphorst GP, Dewey WC (1979) Cell killing and the sequencing of hyperthermia and radiation. Int J Radiat Oncol Biol Phys 5:343–347

Sapozink MD, Deschner EE, Hahn EW (1973) Induction of mitotic synchrony by intermittent hyperthermia in Ehrlich carcinoma in vivo. Nature 244:299–300

Sapozink MD, Gibbs FA Jr, Gates KS, Stewart JR (1984) Regional hyperthermia in the treatment of clinically advanced deep-seated malignancy: results of a study employing an annular array applicator. Int J Radiat Oncol Biol Phys 10:775–776

Schams D, Stephan E, Hooley RD (1980) The effect of heat exposure on blood serum levels of anterior pituitary hormones in calves, heifers, and bulls. Acta Endocrinol (Copenh) 94:309–314

Schlessinger MJ (1986) Heat shock proteins: the search for functions. J Cell Biol 103:321

Schonbaum E, Lomax P (eds) (1990) Thermoregulation physiology and biochemistry. Pergamon, New York, pp 1–506

Schrek R (1966) Sensitivity of normal and leukemic lymphocytes and leukemic myeloblasts to heat. JCI 37:649–654

Schrek R, Stefani SS (1981) Effects of alcohol and hyperthermia on normal and leukemic lymphocytes. Oncology 38:69–71

Schuette WH, Lees DE, Bull JM, Kim YD, Whang-Peng J, Smith R, Tipton HW (1980) Regulation of core body temperature during whole body hyperthermia by oesophageal temperature feedback. Med Biol Eng Comput 18:299–302

Seigel RA, Feldman S, Conforti N, Ben-David M, Chowers I (1979) PRL and ACTH secretion following acute heat exposure, in intact and in hypothalamic deafferentated male rats. Brain Res 778:459–466

Senapati N, Houchens D, Ovejera A, Beard R, Nines R (1982) Ultrasonic hyperthermia and drugs as therapy for human tumor xenografts. Cancer Treat Rep 66:1635–1639

Selker RG, Jacobs SA, Stoller R, Kristojik M, Randall M (1983) On the limits of human tolerance to whole body hyperthermia and simultaneous chemotherapy. Radiat Res 94:550

Shah SA, Dickson JA (1978a) Effect of hyperthermia on the immune response of normal rabbits. Cancer Res 38:3518–3522

Shah SA, Dickson JA (1978b) Effect of hyperthermia on the immunocompetence of VS2 tumor-bearing rabbits. Cancer Res 38:3523–3531

Shen R, Hornback NB, Shidnia H, Shupe RE, Brahmi Z (1987) Whole body hyperthermia decreases lung metastases in lung tumor-bearing mice, possibly via a mechanism involving natural killer cells. J Clin Immunol 7:246–253

Shen R, Hornback NB, Shidnia H, Lu L, Broxmeyer HE, Brahmi Z (1988) Effect of whole body hyperthermia and cyclophosphamide on natural killer cell activity in murine erythroleukemia. Cancer Res 48:4561–4563

Shen R, Hornback NB, Shidnia H, Wu B, Lu L, Broxmeyer HE (1991) Whole body hyperthermia: a potent radioprotector in vivo. Int J Radiat Oncol Biol Phys 20:525–530

Shimm D, Cetas T, Hynynen K, Buechler D, Anhalt D, Aristizabal S, Sykes H, Cassady J (1989) The CDRH helix: clinical thermal dosimetry. Am J Clin Oncol 12:110–113

Shingleton WW, Bryan FA Jr, O'Quinn WL, Kreuger LC (1962) Selective heating and cooling of tissue in cancer chemotherapy. Ann Surg 156:408–416

Shoulder HS, Turner EL, Scott LD (1942) Observations on the results of combined fever and x-ray therapy in the treatment of malignancy. South Med J 35:966–970

Silvestrini B, Hahn GM, Cioli V, Demartino C (1983) Effects of lonidamine alone or combined with hyperthermia in some experimental cell and tumor systems. Br J Cancer 47:221–231

Sim DA, Dewhirst MW, Oleson JR, Grochowski KJ (1984) Estimating the therapeutic advantage of adequate heat. In: Overgaard J (ed) Hyperthermia oncology, vol 1. Taylor and Francis, London, pp 359–362

Skeen MJ, Olkowski ZL, Dupre JR, McLaren JR (1983) Mitogenesis in human lymphocytes following brief exposure to hyperthermia. Int J Radiat Oncol Biol Phys 9:61–66

Slade MS, Simmons RL, Yunis E, Greenberg LJ (1975) Immunodepression after major surgery in normal patients. Surgery 78:363–372

Sladen A, Guntupalli K, Selker R, Weinstock E, Wilks D, Klain M (1981) Hemodynamic responses to induce total body hyperthermia. Clin Res 31:260

Song WC (1984) Effect of local hyperthermia on blood flow and microenvironment: a review. Cancer Res 44:4721s–4730s

Sonigo P, Alizon M, Staskus K, Klatzmann D, Cole S, Danos O, Retzel E, Tiollais P, Haase A, Wain-Hobson S (1985) Nucleotide sequence of the visna lentivirus: relationship to the AIDS virus. Cell 42:369

Sorrell JF (1980) Intravenous lidocaine: an adjunct for nitrous oxide thiopental anesthesia. J Am Assoc Nurse Anesth 48:477–481

Spencer TL, Lehninger AL (1976) L-lactate transport in Erlich ascites tumour cells. Biochem J 154:405–414

Spire B, Dormont D, Barre-Sinoussi F, Montangier L, Chermann JC (1985) Inactivation of lymphadenopathy-associated virus by heat, gamma rays and ultraviolet light. Lancet 152:400–403

Stanley SK, Bressler PB (1990) Heat shock induction of HIV production from chronically infected promonocytic T cell lines. J Immunol 145:1120–1126

Steeves RA, Robins HI, Miller K, Shecterle L, Dennis W (1982) Is the concept of thermal tolerance relevant to whole body hyperthermia (WBH)? Int J Radiat Oncol Biol Phys 8:1845

Steeves RA, Severson SB, Paliwal BR, Anderson S, Robins HI (1986) Matched pair analysis of response to local hyperthermia and megavoltage electron therapy for superficial human tumors. Endocur Ther Hypertherm Oncol 2:163–170

Steeves RA, Robins HI, Miller K, Martin P, Shecterle L, Dennis W (1987) Interaction of whole-body hyperthermia and irradiation in the treatment of AKR mouse leukemia. Int J Radiat Biol 52:935–947

Stehlin JS, Giovanella BC, de Ipolyi PD, Muerz LR, Anderson RF (1975) Results of hyperthermic perfusions for melanoma of the extremities. Surg Gynecol Obstet 140:339–348

Stewart FA, Denekamp J (1977) Sensitization of mouse skin to x-irradiation by moderate heating. Radiology 123:195–200

Stewart FA, Denekamp J (1978) The therapeutic advantage of combined heat and x-rays on a mouse fibrosarcoma. Br J Radiol 51:307–316

Stewart JR, Gibbs FA (1984) Hyperthermia in the treatment of cancer, perspectives on its promise and its problems. Cancer 54:2823–2830

Stewart JR, Gibbs FA Jr, Sapozink MD, Gates KS (1984) Regional hyperthermia using an annular phased array system: preliminary patient and thermometry data. Front Radiat Ther Oncol 18:103–107

Storm FK, Harrison WH, Elliott RS, Hatgetheofilous C, Morton DL (1979a) Human hyperthermia therapy: relationship between tumor type and capacity to induce hyperthermia by radiofrequency. Am J Surg 138:170–174

Storm FK, Harrison WH, Elliott RS, Morton DL (1979b) Normal tissue and solid tumor effects of hyperthermia in animal models and clinical trials. Cancer Res 39:2245–2251

Storm FK, Elliott RS, Harrison WH, Kaiser LR, Morton DL (1981) Radiofrequency hyperthermia of advanced human sarcomas. J Surg Oncol 17:91–98

Strauss AA (1969) Immunologic resistance to carcinoma produced by electrocoagulation. Based on 57 years of experimental and clinical results. Thomas, Springfield

Streffer C (ed) (1978) Cancer therapy by hyperthermia and radiation. Urban and Schwarzenberg, Baltimore

Sultan MF, Tompkins WAF, Cain CA (1984) Inhibition of capping of antigen-antibody complexes on the surface of normal mouse B-lymphocytes by hyperthermia. J Therm Biol 9:193–197

Suit HD, Swayder M (1974) Hyperthermia: potential as an antitumor agent. Cancer 34: 122–129

Szczepanski L, Trott KR (1981) The combined effect of bleomycin and hyperthermia on the adenocarcinoma 284 of the C3H mouse. Eur J Cancer Clin Oncol 17:997–1000

Tapazoglou E, Robins HI, Cohen J, Khatana A, Schmitt CL, Franken K, Corry P, Sapareto SA (1988) The enhancement of cytotoxicity of carboplatin (CBDCA) by whole body hyperthermia (WBH) in the murine AKR leukemia. Proc Am Assoc Cancer Res 29:1342 (abstract)

Teicher BA, Lazo JS, Sartorelli AC (1981a) Classification of antineoplastic agents by their selective toxicities toward oxygenated and hypoxic tumor cells. Cancer Res 41:73–81

Teicher BA, Kowal KA, Sartorelli AC (1981b) Enhancement by hyperthermia of the in vitro cytotoxicity of mitomycin C toward hypoxic tumor cells. Cancer Res 41:1096–1099

Thrall DE, Page RL, Dewhirst MW, Meyer RE, Hoopes PJ, Kornegay JN (1986) Temperature measurements in normal and tumor tissue of dogs undergoing whole body hyperthermia. Cancer Res 46:6229–6235

Thrall DE, Page RL, McLeod DA (1987) Use of insulation to reduce extremity temperature nonuniformity during whole body hyperthermia in dogs. Cancer Res 47:5880–5882

Thrall DE, Dewhirst MW, Samulski TV, Page RL, McLeod DA, Oleson JR (1989a) Temperatures in solid tumors during whole body hyperthermia (WBH) alone and in combination with local hyperthermia (LH). Radiat Res Soc, NAHG abstract Ae-5, p 11

Thrall DE, Page RL, Dewhirst MW, Macy DW, McLeod DA, Scott RJ, Allen S, Gillette EL (1989b) Whole body hyperthermia in dogs using a radiant heating device: effect of surface cooling on temperature uniformity. Int J Hyperthermia 5:137–143

Thrall DE, Dewhirst MW, Page RL, Samulski TV, McLeod DA, Oleson JR (1990) A comparison of temperatures in canine solid tumours during local and whole-body hyperthermia administered alone and simultaneously. Int J Hyperthermia 6:305–317

Thrall DE, Gillette EL, Dewey WC (1975) Effect of heat and ionizing radiation on normal and neoplastic tissues of the C3H mouse. Radiat Res 63:363–377

Thuning CA, Bakir NA, Warren J (1980) Synergistic effect of combined hyperthermia and a nitrosourea in treatment of a murine ependymoblastoma. Cancer Res 40:2726–2729

Tomasovic SP, Turner GN, Dewey WC (1978) Effect of hyperthermia on nonhistone proteins isolated with DNA. Radiat Res 73:535–552

Tompkins WAF, Rama Rao GV, Pantasatos P, Cain CA (1981) Hyperthermia enhancement of antibody-complement cytotoxicity for human colon tumor cells. JNCI 66:453–459

Twentyman PR, Morgan JE, Donaldson J (1978) Enhancement by hyperthermia of the effect of BCNU against the EMT6 mouse tumor. Cancer Treat Rep 62:439–443

Urano M (1986) Kinetics of thermotolerance in normal and tumor tissues: a review. Cancer Res 46:474–482

Urano M, Kim MS (1983) Effect of hyperglycemia in thermochemotherapy of a spontaneous murine fibrosarcoma. Cancer Res 43:3041–3044

Urano M, Rice L, Epstein R, Suit HD, Chu AM (1983) Effect of whole body hyperthermia on cell survival, metastasis frequency, and host immunity in moderately and weakly immunogenic murine tumors. Cancer Res 43:1039–1043

Urano M, Kahn J, Kenton LA (1988) Effect of bleomycin on murine tumor cells at elevated temperatures and two different pH values. Cancer Res 48:615–619

Van der Zee J, Van Rhoon GC, Wike-Hooley JL, Faithfull NS, Reinhold HS (1983) Whole-body hyperthermia in cancer therapy: a report of a phase I–II study. Eur J Cancer Clin Oncol 19:1189–1200

Van der Zee J, Faithfull NS, van Rhoon GC, Reinhold HS (1987) Whole body hyperthermia as a treatment modality. In: Field SB, Franconi C (eds) Physics and technology of hyperthermia. Nijhoff, Boston, pp 420–440

Van der Zee J, van Rhoon GC, Faithfull NS, van den Berg AP (1990) Clinical hyperthermia practice: whole body hyperthermia. In. Field SB, Hand JW (eds) An introduction to the practical aspects of clinical hyperthermia. Taylor and Francis, London, pp 185–212

Van Rijn J, van den Berg J, Schamhart DHJ, van Wijk R (1984) Morphological response and survival of hepatoma cells during fractionated hyperthermia: effect of glycerol. Radiat Res 98:471–478

Van Rhoon GC, Van der Zee J (1983) Cerebral temperature and epidural pressure during whole body hyperthermia in dogs. Res Exp Med 183:47–54

Vose BM, Moudgil GC (1976) Postoperative depression of antibody-dependent lymphocyte cytotoxicity following minor surgery and anesthesia. Immunolgy 30:123–128

Versteegh PMR, van den Hoogen RHWM, Zwaveling A (1981) Systemic hyperthermia by the immersion bath method. Neth J Surg 33:195–199

Wallner KE, Li GC (1987) Effect of drug exposure duration and sequencing on hyperthermic potentiation of mitomycin-C and cisplatin. Cancer Res 47:493–495

Wallner KE, DeGregorio MW, Li GC (1986) Hyperthermic potentiation of cis-diamminedichloroplatinum (II) cytotoxicity in Chinese hamster ovary cells resistant to the drug. Cancer Res 46:6242–6245

Wallner KE, Banda M, Li GC (1987) Hyperthermic enhancement of cell killing by mitomycin C in mitomycin C-resistant Chinese hamster ovary cells. Cancer Res 47:1308–1312

Ward JF (1981) Some biochemical consequences of the spacial distribution of ionizing radiation-produced free radicals. Radiat Res 86:185–195

Warren SL (1935) Preliminary study of the effect of artificial fever upon hopeless tumor cases. Am J Roentgenol Radium Ther 33:75–87

Warters RL, Lyons BW, Axtell-Bartlett J (1987) Inhibition of repair of radiation-induced DNA damage by thermal shock in Chinese hamster ovary cells. Int J Radiat Biol 51:505–517

Weatherburn H (1988) Hyperthermia and AIDS treatment. Br J Radiol 61:862–863

Webb P (1973) Rewarming after diving in cold water. Aerospace Med 44:1152–1157

West KW, Weber TR, Grosfeld JL (1980) Synergistic effect of hyperthermia, papaverine, and chemotherapy in murine neuroblastoma. J Pediatr Surg 15:913–917

Westermark N (1927) The effect of heat upon rat tumors. Scand Arch Physiol 52:257–322

Westra A, Dewey WC (1971) Variation in sensitivity to heat shock during cell cycle of Chinese hamster cells in vitro. Int J Radiat Biol 19:467–477

Whang-Peng J, Lees DE, Schuette WH, Smith R, Bull JM, DeVita VT Jr (1981) Erythrocyte osmotic fragility in patients receiving hyperthermia with and without chemotherapy. Cancer Treat Rep 65:1103

Wickstrom P, Ruiz E, Lilja GP, Hinterkopf JP, Haglin JJ (1976) Accidental hypothermia: core rewarming with partial bypass. Am J Surg 131:622–625

Wiedmeyer J, Hank J, Sondel P, Robins HI (1983) In vitro proliferative responses following whole body hyperthermia. Abstract, Mid-West Autumn Immunology Conference, Chicago, November 2

Wile AG, Nahabedian MY, Plumley DA, Guilmette JE, Mason GR (1983a) Experimental hyperthermic isolation-perfusion using cis-diamminedichloroplatinum (II). Cancer Res 43:3108–3111

Wile AG, Nahabedian MY, Mason GR (1983b) Enhanced tumor growth in experimental whole body hyperthermia. J Surg Oncol 24:119–123

Wilke AV, Jenkins C, Milligan AJ, Legendre A, Frazier DL (1991) Effect of hyperthermia on normal tissue toxicity and on adriamycin pharmacokinetics in dogs. Cancer Res 51:1680–1683

Williams AE, Galt JM (1978) Whole body hyperthermia and immunological function in rats. In: Streffer C, van Beuningen D, Dietzel F et al. (eds) Cancer therapy by hyperthermia and radiation. Urban and Schwarzenberg, Baltimore, pp 294–296

Wondergem J, Strebel FR, Siddik ZH, Newman RA, Bull JMC (1988) The effects of anaesthetics on cisplatinum-induced toxicity at normal temperatures and during whole-body hyperthermia: the influence of NaCl concentration of the vehicle. Int J Hyperthermia 4:643–654

Wright GL (1976) Critical thermal maximum in mice. J Appl Physiol 40:683–687

Yang SJ, Rafla S (1985) Temperature effect on mitoxantrone cytotoxicity in Chinese hamster cells in vitro. Cancer Res 45:3593–3597

Yang HK, Cain CA, Lockwood, Tompkins WAF (1983) Effects of microwave exposure on the hamster immune system. 1. Natural killer cell activity. Bioelectromagnetics 4:123–139

Yatvin MB (1977) The influence of membrane liquid composition and procaine on hyperthermic death of cells. Int J Radiat Biol 32:513–521

Yatvin MB (1988) An approach to AIDS therapy using hyperthermia and membrane modification. Med Hypotheses 27:163–165

Yatvin MB, Clifton KH, Dennis WH (1979) Hyperthermia and local anesthetics: potentiation of survival in tumor-bearing mice. Science 205:195–196

Yatvin MB, Schmitz BJ, Rusy BF, Dennis WH (1980) Local anesthetic alteration of cell survival after hyperthermia or irradiation. In: Fink R (ed) Molecular mechanisms of anesthesia, progress in anesthesia, vol 2. Raven, New York, pp 495–499

Yau TM (1979) Procaine-mediated modification of membranes and the response to x-irradiation and hyperthermia in mammalian cells. Radiat Res 80:523–541

Yerushalmi A (1976) Influence on metastatic spread of whole body or local tumor hyperthermia. Exp J Cancer 12:455–463

Yerushalmi A (1978) Combined treatment of a solid tumour by local hyperthermia and actinomycin D. Br J Cancer 37:827–832

Yerushalmi A, Hazan G (1979) Control of Lewis lung carcinoma by combined treatment with local hyperthermia and cyclophosphamide: preliminary results. Isr J Med Sci 15:462–463

Zanker KS, Lange J (1982) Whole body hyperthermia and natural killer cell activity. Lancet 1:1079–1080

Zarling JM, Kung PC (1980) Monoclonal antibodies which distinguish between human NK cells and cytotoxic T-lymphocytes. Nature 288:394–396

Subject Index

Clinical Thermology

Subseries Thermotherapy

Series Editor: M. Gautherie

Biological Basis of Oncologic Thermotherapy

Methods of External Heating

Methods of Hyperthermia Control

Thermal Dosimetry and Treatment Planning

Whole-Body Hyperthermia:
Biological and Clinical Aspects

Interstitial, Endocavitary and Perfusional Hyperthermia – Methods and Clinical Trials